THE
CLINICAL SUCCESS FORMULA

How to Reduce Anxiety, Build Confidence, and Pass with Flying Colors

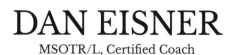

DAN EISNER

MSOTR/L, Certified Coach

PRAISE FOR THE CLINICAL SUCCESS FORMULA

"If you're looking for easy to follow guidance on how to maximize performance in the clinic, you will definitely want to add *The Clinical Success Formula* to your library. Dan has taken his years of experience in many healthcare settings and generously offers practical strategies for enhancing the quality of service you provide. I found myself relaxing more with each page, as the book includes countless jewels of wisdom that are helpful both personally and professionally. He shows you how to easily transform the emotions of fear and anxiety into acceptance and compassion, and how you can consistently access your greatest intelligence – your intuition. Even though this book will help you to succeed clinically, Dan shares skills for a lifetime that will help maximize your potential in all areas of life. I know it is a resource I will continue to reference for years to come."

—Emmy Vadnis, Holistic OT

"This book offers so much more than a formula for students. Any clinician who finds their energy sapped or their self-compassion diminished will benefit from the replenishing philosophy and techniques offered in *The Clinical Success Formula*."

—Hilary Robinson, OTR/L

"As both a healthcare educator and practicing OT, I can say *The Clinical Success Formula* is a must read. I was fortunate to be mentored by Dan when I was a student and beginning my career as a licensed professional. Words cannot describe the empowering and lasting impact that his approach (beautifully refined and summarized in this book) has had on my personal and professional life. I continue to experience the value of this formula in action on a daily basis – it is truly life changing for you and the people you serve. This book will help you to become more self-reliant and comfortable in your own skin; two essential skills for maximizing your performance in all areas of life."

—Laura Cunningham, OTR/L

"*The Clinical Success Formula* is not just for students, it's an excellent resource for all healthcare providers. As a seasoned social worker, I have experienced how easy it can be to forget ourselves while taking care of others. Dan gently reminds us of the importance of treating ourselves with the same level of compassion we give our patients, and he shares a practical road map for providing high quality care."

—Majbritt Jensen, LCSW-C

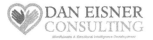

Printed in the United States of America
ISBN: 978-0-9976757-3-3

TABLE OF CONTENTS

FOREWORD

The teachings within *The Clinical Success Formula* are both cutting edge science and age-old, universal knowledge. They offer healthcare professionals and their clients a greater perspective on what it means to be healthy, and how to effectively thrive in work and life.

Neuroscience tells us that we create our personal reality "from thought" based on the attitudes, beliefs, and truths that fit into our evolving understanding of life.

As Dan Eisner so brilliantly shares, the vast majority of our everyday thinking and feeling is subconscious, automatic, and survival-based. When the raging chemicals of survival—which is stress—become the habituated program, it's impossible to truly be in the present moment and to perform at our best. As long as we are living in stress, there will always be a constant struggle.

True success can only be attained by learning how to consciously transcend the "normal" stressed states of being, and to reprogram ourselves to live in a state of inner peace and joy.

How is that achieved?

It's all here in *The Clinical Success Formula*. Dan offers you the exquisite knowledge and practical applications to not only pass your clinical rotations, but to succeed beyond your wildest expectations. My advice is to contemplate and absorb every word, then go out into your life and experiment with its teachings.

—Karin Sokel

Certified NCS Consultant for Dr. Joe Dispenza, NeuroChange Solutions

PREFACE

Why did I write this book? Because I care about your success and the quality of care in our Healthcare System.

I have been inspired and motivated by the realization that the amazing connection I have experienced with countless clients is not the norm, and I don't think it should be that way. I know that given the proper tools all healthcare providers can learn to serve from a much deeper place on a consistent basis.

It used to (and still does to an extent) frustrate me to see people (not *patients*—I think that word should be abolished) being treated in a less than outstanding manner, so I channeled that energy into this book.

Even though I enjoy working with and coaching people directly, I am equally, if not more, passionate about training other professionals to bring more energy, more of themselves, into their practice.

My goal is that you find something here that works for you to pass your clinical rotations with flying colors, build good habits from the start, and become the successful healthcare professional of your dreams.

INTRODUCTION

Maya Angelou said, "People won't remember what you did, but they will always remember how you made them feel." As a professional, it is important to be competent in your area of expertise. Your capacity and skill, however, are not necessarily going to make the people you serve feel good or trust you.

We all want to feel understood, respected, and be treated like human beings, especially when stuck in the role of being a patient.

After working for nearly 20 years in the healthcare field, I can tell you that being treated like a human being is *not* the norm in our healthcare system. The reason is that we place high value on time, efficiency, and productivity. Humanity, as a state of being, has kind of become an inconvenience, like we don't have the time to be kind or to give one another our fullest attention. We get so identified with our roles (nurse, therapist, doctor, etc.), and the to-dos they require, that we have essentially become "human doings," which is reflected in the depersonalized quality of care that we experience at times.

When we forget who we are behind the roles we play every day as healthcare providers, we cannot possibly see the humanity in our patients. Yet, it truly takes a great deal of courage and openness to discover the subtle ways in which we fall into this trap.

The question is: Are we just doing our jobs mechanically or are we consciously serving real people? Recognizing this subtle but powerful distinction makes all the difference, both for you and for the people you serve.

You Are Not a Healthcare Professional

My good friend Laura is an occupational therapy (OT) professor at Elizabethtown College. The first thing she teaches is, "You are *not* an occupational therapist," which evokes a number of blank, confused stares from her students.

She wants them to understand that being an OT is not their identity. If they do not sense their own humanity, they will not recognize it in their patients, who deserve to be treated with understanding, care, and respect.

Personally, I am blessed to work with awesome, passionate people who provide great care. But there are many healthcare professionals who have not yet learned this priceless lesson and remain solely identified with their role. They cannot and do not fully appreciate the humanness within the patients they are treating.

I say this without any judgment, recognizing that everyone is doing the best they can from their present state of consciousness (Deepak Chopra). However, I believe that we can all be better role models for the people we are serving.

Consider this: Why did you choose a career in healthcare?

You're probably saying (just like the rest of us in the field), "I want to help people." We all know, on some level, that this is not the entire truth. Secretly, some of us want to help others so we can feel better about ourselves. Thinking this way is dangerous because it is so easy to forget the importance of self-care in the process.

I thought this way for years and did not realize how hypocritical I was. I was teaching the importance of wellness from a place of imbalance. Instead of developing a healthier sense of balance by taking care of myself, I was secretly trying to get my fix by helping others. This, of course, left me feeling progressively more dissatisfied. Something had to give.

After years of struggle, I finally learned that nothing is more important than my personal growth and well-being. Ironically, these are the fundamentals of high-quality healthcare.

Even though I am still doing the same work I have done for years, the focus has shifted dramatically. I am now my highest priority. This may sound selfish, but I assure you, it is not. Why do pilots announce, "In case of emergency, put on your own mask first"? We cannot save anyone without first attending to our own needs.

Today, I regularly receive inspired comments from clients. I don't say this to toot my own horn but to illustrate how much more powerful we can be by making our own self-care a priority.

In the context of teaching many of the principles in this book, I frequently ask my clients, "Is the way that I'm approaching you different from what you normally get? How is it different?"

"Oh my God, *yes*, it is different!" is the typical response, followed by these types of comments:

"You're not talking *at* me; this is more of a discussion we are having."

"This feels *real*."

"You're treating me like a person, not a patient."

"You're so calm, and you put me at ease."

"I can tell you're not just lecturing from a book."

Comments like these indicate that I am focused on my deepest intentions, so they are nice to hear but I no longer take them personally (i.e., "Look what I did!"). I have learned, and continue to learn, that looking for external validation is a losing battle; we can *never* get enough.

I also received great comments when I was consumed by my therapist role. They would provide a momentary boost of energy, but then I would need something else to fill the void I was feeling from focusing on surface intentions. I was living in fear, never knowing where or how I was going to get my next fix.

I had put off writing this book for a long time, but I was not aware of the reason until recently. It is now painfully obvious to me why I delayed this task.

I was TERRIFIED of failure!

What if I cannot do it?

What if people will not like it?

What if no one will want to buy it?

You get the idea.

Do I want to make a difference in the quality of care in our healthcare system? Absolutely, but that is no longer my top priority.

My primary intention is to enjoy the process of writing this book, not for some future result but for the process of writing it. If I write it from a place of fear and from being too concerned about how the book will be received, then I am not practicing what I preach. And that defeats everything I am doing.

My secondary intention is to support other healthcare providers in learning how to practice better self-care, because everyone, providers and patients, wins in the process.

As you embark on your clinical rotations, I understand that you have an important goal in mind—namely, to pass and become a licensed professional. I am inviting you to take a different approach to creating a successful clinical rotation and productive healthcare career. I would like you to experience self-care as the foundation of providing quality healthcare to others. Making **you** the top priority is the recipe for your success as a healthcare professional.

I believe this book is the best CliffsNotes-type book on personal growth and clinical success ever created. You may want to deepen your understanding by exploring some of the additional resources I recommend but, I assure you, this book is self-contained. It utilizes the most essential pieces of the puzzle and the practical applications of everything you need to know in order to facilitate your personal and professional success.

I've organized the bulk of the material using a computer-type model: Programming Yourself for Clinical Success. Each chapter is designed to expand your knowledge base, and the recommended techniques and exercises will help to deepen your understanding.

The chapters share a common theme, which is to help you become more present (in the zone) in your life. Honestly, can you think of anything more valuable?

Treating the Person, Not the Patient

A few years ago, a new graduate joined our department. She was young, smart, driven, and ready to make a difference. Clearly she had the technical and intellectual understanding required to be a great healthcare provider. However, by her own admission, she also came in with a chip on her shoulder (disguised anxiety). She was initially quite guarded and rigid and presented an attitude of "I already know what I'm doing, and I don't need anyone's help."

Even though she was initially resistant to many of the ideas covered in this book, she couldn't help but notice that the clients found them helpful. She progressively became more open and started asking questions.

One day, I invited her to observe a one-on-one treatment with a severely depressed client. It turned out to be an amazing session—the woman (the client) transformed right in front of our eyes.

After the session, I asked the new graduate, "Do you see (understand) now?" She replied, "Oh my God."

She spent that evening writing down her thoughts and making the connection with her behaviors. She was astounded at what she began to learn about herself, and she began to experience the value of making self-awareness a priority. At first, she only noticed how it was impacting her personally, but shortly thereafter, a patient gave her some feedback that she will never forget.

The patient, a man with paranoid schizophrenia, was admitted to her unit. He was extremely guarded and unwilling to speak to anyone, but this young graduate had a great conversation with him. After the session, he told her, "I usually don't tell people anything, but the moment I saw you, I knew you were here with me."

Her presence cut right through his illness and brought out the very best in him. Imagine how different our healthcare system could be if all providers operated this way.

A few years ago, I gave a guest lecture at Ohio State University that included many of the ideas you will discover in this book. The lecture was generally well received, but I was shocked (and so was Dr. Cleary, professor and clinical coordinator of the School of Health and Rehabilitation Sciences) to see that many of the students could not recognize the connection between the material presented, which revolved around self-awareness and attention, and being successful on their rotations.

In retrospect, though, I get it. I spent years of my life focused on end goals, saying things like, "I just want to pass!" I paid little attention to the process that would facilitate this desired outcome. Even though I was "successful," that is, I passed, I would stress, being too concerned about the end result and the fear of failing. Today, I am a lot wiser.

A friend (also a healthcare professional) was a successful college tennis player, winning the championship four years in a row. Yet, she quit after spending those four years stressing about—winning. Yes, she was a winner, but was she truly successful?

True success has everything to do with being balanced. Being too relaxed and unfocused can lead to inefficiency and lack of productivity. Hyper-focused attention, on the other hand, can tax the brain and body, putting both into a fight-or-flight mode. Either behavior can lead to difficulty.

I think we healthcare professionals can agree that being too relaxed and unfocused is not how we would describe the typical behavior of those aspiring to a career in this field. They probably wouldn't be in either of those states unless there was good reason.

After working in the healthcare field for close to 20 years, I can tell you that healthcare professionals being hyper-focused, and sometimes downright neurotic, is a much more common problem than one thinks.

And now, to you, the healthcare professional.

This book is written for you. While many of the subjects covered may not seem directly related to your success in clinical rotations, I'm going to ask you to take a leap of faith and trust me.

What you will learn here is intimately connected to your own clinical success and to becoming a true healer in life.

If you are feeling a bit skeptical, thinking, "This isn't about my rotation, this is about *me*, and it is not going to help me pass," consider the following questions: Will being more relaxed while maintaining focus help my performance? Will learning how to manage my emotions (e.g., anxiety, fear) boost my confidence? Will learning how to stay "in the zone" help me be successful? Will being able to connect with the people I am serving help me do well?

If you answered yes to all of the above (I can't imagine that you did not), then put aside your preconceptions about achieving success on your rotations and immerse yourself in this book. Specific strategies and techniques to handle common challenges will be addressed, but mostly you will learn about what I call the "roadmap to your own wisdom."

People often ask me how they should do "X" (lots of options as fill-ins). My general response is, "I don't know how you should do that because there are too many dynamics involved for me to tell you exactly what to do. But I promise that if you learn how to stay internally focused and connected to the greater part of your identity (i.e., being in the zone), you'll just *know* what to do and you'll do it."

This book is not really about answering specific questions related to clinical success. It is about learning how to access your own answers naturally.

Years ago, a family friend asked me, "Can you help Alex prepare for his medical school interviews?" I said, "Yes, but it's not about the interviews. If Alex knows how to show up as Alex, just being himself and not needing to impress anyone, then he'll do well."

He did well and has since become one of those unique physicians who makes their own self-care a priority.

Now it's your turn. So let's get started by clarifying and polishing your intentions as you embark on your clinical rotations.

The Power of Intention

One of my favorite teachers, Tara Brach (www.tarabrach.com), deepened my understanding of the power of intention. She reminded me that every thought we have carries an energy or intention that creates karma.

As you will learn in this book, we are often not truly aware of our thoughts and intentions and thus create negative karma by "default," or lack of attention.

Consider the following:

When I am rushing through traffic or just speeding mindlessly, what is my intention?

Clearly, my primary intention is to get to where I am going as fast as possible. I am making *getting there* more important than my own safety. While this may seem obvious, the reality is that the most important things in life (safety, being true to oneself, etc.) tend to become secondary.

Imagine how many accidents could be prevented if we stopped for a moment before driving and set a very clear primary intention of getting to our destination in a safe and peaceful manner.

Now, I'd like to invite you to get clear about your deepest intentions as you prepare for your clinical rotations. Pause and think.

I put off writing this book for a long time because of the fear I created in myself. I was hyper-focused on the intention to **sell a lot of books and help people!**

I certainly would like to experience those results, but is that my deepest intention?

Surface intentions, like "selling a lot of books" or "passing my clinical," create undue stress from the fear of not reaching the goal. And, like drugs, they only result in fleeting karma highs. My college tennis-player friend is a good example. She made *winning* more important than herself. So, even when she won, she was never really satisfied.

It is very easy to operate unconsciously from surface intentions like these as you enter into your clinical rotations.

Surface Intentions for Clinical Success

Common examples of surface intentions include:

"I just want to pass."

"I want to impress my supervisor."

"I want to help people."

I'm not suggesting that these intentions are bad, but they do not point to our highest priorities. For example, "I want to help people" is a surface intention that may secretly mean, "I want to help people so I can feel better about myself." No one wants to become dependent on external conditions to feel good internally. Surface intentions do not take this truth into account.

Think about your deepest intentions right now, and keep them in the forefront of your mind. Even though I am clear about writing this book for the purpose of writing this book, I can still sense those surface intentions trying to take over at times. I would be in a constant state of stress if I were not committed to reminding myself of my deepest intentions on a regular basis.

Here are a few examples of deep intentions you may want to consider, or feel free to create your own list.

Deepest Intentions for Clinical Success

My intention is to put forward my absolute best effort and trust that I will do well.

My intention is to impress myself by overcoming whatever challenges may arise.

My intention is to be the greatest role model that I can be for the people I am serving.

Paying close attention to your deepest intentions is the best way to ensure your external success (passing, impressing, helping, etc.), while fully enjoying and appreciating the experience.

The Over-Achiever with Low Self-Esteem

Several years ago, I supervised an outstanding OT student. She was smart, but open-minded. She asked questions and accepted feedback well and didn't expect her hand to be held. She was also very creative and not afraid to experiment with innovative ways of providing care. She was a delightful person. In fact, we hired her after she graduated.

During her 12-week clinical rotation, she posed a fun question of the day to our staff during lunches. One day, the question was, "What's something about yourself that you want to improve?"

I was shocked to hear her answer, "I'd like to have better self-esteem." I thought, How could she not have high self-esteem? She was a "rock star" of a student.

As you already know, the only thing that ultimately matters is how we feel about ourselves. The great things we accomplish in life (like this student had) really have very little internal value (i.e., they don't raise self-esteem) when we lose sight of our deepest intentions. She was having an amazing impact on the people around her, yet she still didn't feel good about herself. I don't know about you, but I can relate to this experience.

The last piece of advice I offered her was, "You are already **awesome**. Please understand that you don't have to prove that to yourself or anyone. You do the things that you do because *you are already great*, not so that you can be great someday in the future."

This subtle distinction makes all the difference in the world, and is an important reminder of the power of intention.

CHAPTER 1

EMBRACING FEAR

If you are like most aspiring healthcare professionals, the thought of "What if I fail my clinical?" probably crosses your mind way too often. If you are feeling ashamed about this, then here is what you have to do: STOP IT!

Stop it?

Yes. Stop feeling ashamed about the fear of failing. It is a legitimate concern. You have spent an enormous amount of time, energy, and money educating yourself to become a licensed professional. The reality is that you cannot graduate and set off on your career if you don't pass your clinical rotations.

So, how could you *not* be scared of failing?

Ironically, I highly doubt that fear causes many students to fail. But fear can be damaging in a different way. An occupational therapy student once told me, "I was so scared of failing my first clinical that I didn't do a very good job. I got through it, but it wasn't easy."

She passed. But was she really "successful"?

Many students equate not failing with success. But that's a very limited definition that leads professionals to a less than optimal performance.

I define clinical success this way:

Clinical success means completing the requirements in an

emotionally balanced state while feeling great about yourself and about the difference you are making in the lives of the people you serve.

Fear that is not managed properly will definitely prevent true clinical success. Yet fear is completely normal, and even healthy, when it is accepted and properly channeled into preparing for any "scary" endeavor.

No One Cares about Your Grades

Clinical rotations are the pinnacle experience of your education. You now have to put it all together and make it work in the real world. The rotations mark the transition from student to independent working professional. It's certainly an exciting time, but it can also be a very challenging one.

Clinical success requires a great deal more than book smarts. Your grade point average does not mean anything when it comes to providing quality healthcare. It is your ability to manage all the dynamics (caseload, time management, performance anxiety, etc.) that will enable you to perform at your highest level, not your As and Bs.

Here are just a few of the potential challenges you may encounter.

1. How to manage performance anxiety.
2. How to manage the student/supervisor relationship.
3. How to manage time and caseload.
4. How to work with unmotivated patients.
5. How to establish and maintain relationships with the healthcare team.
6. How to manage constructive feedback.

7. How to maintain a healthy work/life balance.

8. How to manage emotionally challenged clients.

9. How to connect to culturally diverse clients.

10. How to trust the therapeutic process (not trying to control/be perfect).

The primary responsibility of a healthcare education is to teach the scientific and technical aspects. It is not designed as a program to teach you how to manage your emotions, which is the key to handling challenges.

Being familiar with common techniques and strategies for handling all of the above mentioned is very useful, but there are far too many dynamics in any situation to provide clear-cut solutions that are 100% effective (which is what typical neurotic healthcare students want!). Infinite potential solutions exist, but where you stand emotionally is what will determine your best course of action in any given moment.

Most of us, however, are unaware of our emotions. We do not recognize the subtle ways in which they distract our attention and influence our choices. Our addiction to multitasking points to this truth. Many people actually consider multitasking to be an essential skill. Yes, externally we need to manage a variety of activities at once. But what happens when we multitask "internally"?

Consider the following examples: How do you feel when you are in the shower thinking about school? How do you feel when working on a paper while worrying about your grade? How do you feel when you are doing a task while worrying about the outcome?

You don't need to be Freud to recognize the damaging effects of internal multitasking. Without question it causes a great deal of internal chaos that limits our performance. Unconscious emotions run wild, like the rat-on-the-wheel in the human mind.

I love asking clients, "Do you know what it's like to be in the zone?" They usually perk up and say, "Oh yeah, it's great. I'm not even really thinking, I'm just focused and at my best."

We love being in the zone because we are relaxed but focused— *fully* in the present moment. It is our lack of self-awareness and limited ability to manage emotions that prevent access to this precious state.

The good news is that you already have *your own* abilities to consistently stay in the zone. And, don't you just *know* what to do when you are in the zone? The answer is yes, and this is because you are accessing your wisdom by fully being in the present moment. What's more, you *can* learn to consistently stay there (in the moment) by practicing what you will learn in this book.

I'm not here to teach you anything new. My intention is to remind you of what you already intuitively know and to provide you with a great road map to optimize your performance. This, of course, will carry over to your life in general.

The best way to start is by working through your own "blocks." Think about this: the importance of *balance*.

Can we expect the people we serve to get on board if we are not equally committed?

You know the answer. So, commit right now to becoming the greatest role model you can be. The formula I have created will help you tremendously. All you have to do is give it a little attention and energy.

The Formula Works

I spent the first 30 years of my life (I am not exaggerating) in an almost constant state of unease. Then, I took another seven years desperately trying to feel better. I did not realize that I was primarily learning what *does not work* for the first several years after I committed to my own personal growth.

But I don't regret one second of my experience. It has enabled me to condense over 20,000 hours of personal-growth experience into a simple nuts-and-bolts formula that *works*.

Relax, You're Not Supposed to Know Everything

When I was a student, I was convinced that I should know everything before I started. This didn't make any sense, but I wasn't very logical at the time. I was worried about failing, and I wasn't alone in this respect.

I once heard a story about the Dalai Lama's response when he was asked a serious question. He replied with, "I don't know," in a lighthearted way, which elicited a palpable sense of relief in the audience.

The audience felt relief because many of them unconsciously felt pressured to know everything. When the Dalai Lama admitted to not knowing something, he gave everyone else permission to be okay with not knowing everything as well, at least for that moment.

I believe the pressure to "know" is particularly prevalent in healthcare. We are seen as the experts who are supposed to have all the answers. The people we serve have high expectations, and if you're like me, you probably don't want to disappoint them.

However, when we don't have the courage to admit (to ourselves especially) that we don't have all the answers, we forfeit our ability to access new information. The more we get comfortable operating from a place of "I don't know, but I am willing to learn," the more we can access our greatest intelligence—our intuition.

This is exactly what happens when we are providing treatment "in the zone." We are outside the box, immersed in the present moment, accessing the most creative and innovative ways of providing healthcare.

As a student, no one expects you to know everything, and I'd encourage you to relish this fact. Do your best to operate from a place of "I don't know, but I am excited to learn." I promise you, maintaining this attitude will help you relax, making the process of learning much easier.

CHAPTER 2

PROGRAMMING YOURSELF FOR CLINICAL SUCCESS: THE THREE KEYS

Years ago, I introduced many of the ideas covered in this book to a few occupational therapy students. I had never thought about what I do as it relates to clinical success until one of the students said, "This explains how we can best apply ourselves therapeutically. Our teacher was trying to explain it, but this really is it!"

"How do I use these techniques with my patients?" is the most common question asked when I am training healthcare professionals. My answer is always the same: "Use the techniques on yourself, and then you will know how to use them with your patients." The key to clinical success is managing *your own* emotions. It is the foundation for establishing rapport and for helping others maximize their potential.

I have learned a great deal since meeting those students. The most important discovery is that we are clueless when it comes to understanding what I like to call "The Human Operating System."

We simply don't understand how our minds and emotions work, and we try to "fix" ourselves using antiquated knowledge. Einstein stated, "You cannot solve a problem on the same level at which it was created."

Part of our human conditioning is believing that there is something wrong with us, and we have to fix it.

We are not perfect, and we can all benefit from making changes. The problem is that we take this human conditioning so personally. Instead of observing our self-limiting behaviors (overeating, too much social media, etc.) with a sense of compassion, we judge ourselves. This only perpetuates the behavior, making it more difficult to change.

The most common example is substance addiction, the "*I am* an Alcoholic" phenomenon. Even if a person is addicted to alcohol, being an alcoholic is **not** their identity, no matter how much they believe this to be true.

Unconscious identification with emotion and certain behaviors, as opposed to with a substance, are the most prevalent addictions. Common examples include:

"I am a worrier."

"I am a perfectionist."

"I am a people pleaser."

These behaviors are not necessarily bad, but they do become problematic when continuously repeated. Worry, as an example, is not your (or anyone's) real identity. It is just a conditioned habit that can be changed by a commitment to increased self-awareness and behavior modification.

Excessive thinking is the real culprit behind many of our destructive habits. It is an addiction in itself, which is defined as anything you cannot stop doing (Joe Dispenza). Most of us do not see it that way because the behavior is so common; yet, it truly is the root cause of most human suffering (Eckhart Tolle).

I was nearly consumed by negative thinking until my mid-thirties.

I completely personified someone who believed he was broken and needed fixing.

I spent about a decade trying to fix myself before realizing that I was wrong. I now recognize, in a deep, meaningful way, that there is truly nothing wrong with me.

It is one thing to understand this intellectually and quite another to realize this on a deeper, emotional level. I still have my flawed human conditioning, but I no longer take it so personally. This has made the process of change significantly easier.

I always tell my clients, "I don't care what you have done or what diagnosis you have, there is NOTHING wrong with you at your core. And the same is true for everyone else."

The clients who hear this usually shed a few tears because they recognize this truth within themselves. There is nothing wrong with *you* either, no matter how much you (or your environment [family, friends, media, etc.]) tell yourself otherwise.

Even though we are perfect at our core, we all have our "outdated software." So let's talk about how you can begin to upgrade your software for clinical success.

The three keys of Programming Yourself for Clinical Success include a basic understanding of (1) the Human Operating System, (2) Open-Focus Attention, and (3) the Science of Emotion. These topics will be discussed in the following sections. They are like the "software" required for clinical success and include specific areas of knowledge and exercises to help train your brain and body to work more efficiently throughout your clinical rotations.

KEY #1: THE HUMAN OPERATING SYSTEM

"Experience without knowledge is ignorance," says Dr. Joe Dispenza, best-selling author of *Breaking the Habit of Being Yourself*.

Understanding the Human Operating System and how it can empower you is the #1 key to passing your clinical rotations with flying colors. It will promote success in other areas as well. The more you understand exactly how to access the "zone," the better you can use that information to optimize your performance.

Before we begin, I would like to point out that I am going to use several words interchangeably. It will make more sense later on but for now *Energy*, *Consciousness*, *Awareness*, and *Space* all refer to what I call the Human Operating System.

Eckhart Tolle considers these words just "road signs" pointing to something that cannot be fully understood by the rational mind. So please don't despair if you do not understand these concepts yet.

You Are NOT Your Body and You Are NOT Your Mind

The atom is made up of 99.999% empty space and energy (Dispenza, *You Are the Placebo*). Atoms are the building blocks of the human body. This means we are made of more empty space and energy than of flesh and blood. It is difficult for the logical left brain to grasp this truth, but consider for a moment what this really means.

This can be a scary realization because it begs the question, "If I am *not* my mind or body, then who or what am I?"

We live in a materialistic culture. Our sense of self-worth has become distorted. Many of us believe that our identity depends on our attributes and/or possessions, such as improving physical attractiveness, acquiring more or better things, or achieving success.

As a result, we desperately pursue goals (degrees, relationships, money, children, etc.), falsely believing they will provide us with a more desirable identity in the future. The problem is that our external pursuits can become like drugs. We build up a tolerance and progressively need more, until it stops working.

This is the classic over-achiever syndrome, where no amount of success is ever satisfying.

I am not suggesting that pursuing external goals is wrong. But I am saying that our achievements (no matter how great) have nothing to do with our real identity. No amount of success will ever fill the void that comes from getting lost in external pursuits. This is why it is important to start focusing on the greater, internal part of our identity.

Remember, you are *consciousness*, which is another way of saying you are the space in which all things exist (Tolle, *The Power of Now*). Again, don't try to figure this out; no one can understand it intellectually. Deep down, however, you already *know* it to be true.

We Are Not IN the Zone, We ARE the Zone

I ask my clients, "Do you ever notice a part of you that just *knows* what you should do, even though you don't always listen?" (E.g., I *know* I should have worked out, but I stayed on the couch instead.)

The part of us that does not *think* but just *knows* is the true self.

Consider how you think and feel when you are in the zone. Most people say, "I'm not thinking. I'm just focused and I feel great."

What do you think that feeling is?

If you're thinking, "It is the real me," you are correct. The feeling of being in the zone is in fact our true identity. It is *not* a thought, an idea, or a concept but rather the peaceful energy we can sense when we are fully in the moment. We mistakenly believe that external things or activities can produce that feeling, like the following:

1. "My dog makes me feel good."

2. "Art makes me feel good."

3. "Playing basketball makes me feel good."

But I am sure you have noticed that these don't work 100% of the time. So, what is the difference? Why do things that often make us feel good seem ineffective at other times?

It has everything to do with our attention. We feel great when we are in the present moment and stressed when distracted. We enjoy activities, people, or animals but the real, most satisfying element is the "being-ness" of the present moment (Tolle, *Power of Now*).

I often observe clients experiencing profound shifts during our sessions. Frequently, they say the session made them feel better. I always make it clear that it was their *full attention* to the session that produced the positive feeling.

A typical comment may be, "I'm glad that you found our time helpful, but understand that you are feeling better primarily because you chose to fully attend. You don't need me to feel this way. All it takes is a commitment to paying closer attention to what you're doing throughout your day."

The more we attend to the present moment, the better we stay connected to the Human Operating System, our true identity.

Where you place your attention is where you place your energy.

—DR. JOE DISPENZA

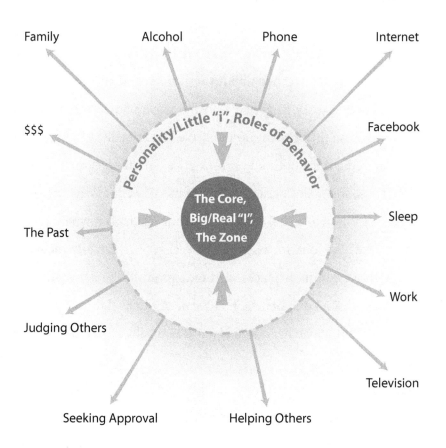

A Picture Is Worth a Thousand Words

Dr. Joe Dispenza uses a variation of the preceding graphic in his workshops. The simplicity and wisdom of what this conveys is quite powerful. Understandably, it is one of the things clients find most helpful.

When we are in the zone, our attention (energy) is directed toward our core, not toward the outcome, which is why we feel and perform at our best. We are permitting the Human Operating System, our true self, to perform its function of guiding the physical self toward the right course of action. And, doesn't it work beautifully when we get out of the way?

The moment we (the physical self) try to take over, our performance suffers. We get too concerned about the results, and the body tenses. We overanalyze and try to get back to the zone, which only takes us further away from the present moment. We lose the ability to adapt, an essential ingredient for optimal performance, and we feel miserable.

When I share this diagram with clients, I ask them where does peace come from? The usual response is from inside. But where do we look for peace? We look for it everywhere else. (I've actually included several of those common places in the diagram.) This is because we have been conditioned to believe that we *need* external things to make us feel better. But all we need to feel good naturally is to focus on our true self.

Our core (the big or real sense of "I") is very solid and strong, but our exterior (physical self, personality, little "i") is very weak. It is like a leaky gas tank, where no amount of "gas" (degrees, money, recognition, etc.) will be enough to fill the unease we feel when we forget about ourselves while pursuing external gratification.

I'm not saying that we should not pursue external gratification. But I do think we should be careful not to do so at the expense of our own well-being. I focused practically all of my energy on external pursuits for years, which caused me to eventually feel indifferent and downright apathetic.

I just didn't care anymore.

About a year and a half ago, my friend and coach Karin asked me a very powerful question after I told her how I was feeling.

"What's your intention?"

I realized, in a deep and profound way, that I was making my goals more important than my self. My intentions were all surface oriented—including helping others, winning money at poker, playing better golf—all for the purpose of temporarily inflating my ego, or false sense of self.

Karin finished our conversation by saying, "You might want to consider upgrading your intention to Joy—make joy your highest priority."

It was a life-changing moment that deepened my understanding of true success. I realized that true success could only be achieved by focusing on the joy of the present moment as we pursue our external goals.

You will discover that it is *not* one or the other—my goals or me—it is **both**, my goals **and** me. Focusing on both is actually much easier in the long run, but it does require a shift in how we pay attention.

We intuitively *know* how to do this because it is precisely how we are focused when in the zone. My favorite resource, *The Open-Focus Brain*, by Dr. Les Fehmi and Jim Robbins, validates that it is a powerful tool for optimizing performance.

LOOKING IN THE MIRROR

The Awareness behind the Diagnosis

No matter what diagnosis a person may have, it's not their identity. This may seem obvious, but the subtle ways in which many of us fall into the identity trap are not always easy to see.

A few years ago, I worked with a guy diagnosed with major depression. I showed him an amusing but powerful *MADtv* skit featuring Bob Newhart as a therapist (you can find it searching for "Bob Newhart, Stop It").

I recommend watching the video to see "Dr. Newhart" deliver his simple and unique approach to therapy. Regardless of his client's issue, he'd just tell him or her to "STOP IT!"

After my client watched the video, he said, "If it was that easy to stop it, I would."

I replied, "You're right. As long as you believe you are this depressed guy, there is very little you can do. But you're not your illness; you are the awareness that knows it exists. Once you start operating from the awareness that is your true identity, you will be able to manage your depression much more effectively."

He ended up doing quite well. In fact, I run into him several times a year, since we work at the same hospital. He's moved forward with his life and now has a new position that he loves. He is also engaged to his girlfriend.

Does he still experience symptoms of depression? My guess is yes, but the frequency and severity of the symptoms have declined significantly. He no longer identifies with his diagnosis. This has enabled him to consistently "STOP IT" and to make the behavioral changes that keep him balanced.

KEY #2: OPEN-FOCUS ATTENTION

Before I get into what Open Focus entails, I would like to share a bit more of my personal history.

I have devoted more than the last 10 years to my personal growth. Even though I progressed during the first seven, I treaded water in more ways than I would like to admit.

I intuitively knew this was happening, but the truth (me struggling) became more difficult to ignore after I consulted with a neurofeedback specialist. Her equipment indicated that I had very high beta brainwave activity, a reflection of my overly analytical and anxiety-ridden mind.

Shortly after that visit, my friend Alex introduced me to Open-Focus Attention. I experienced its value immediately, and it quickly became the most integral part of my self-care practice.

In February 2014, I had my brain mapped by brain expert Dr. Jeffrey Fannin. The results confirmed that I now had healthier brain activity. The high beta brainwave activity detected earlier had diminished considerably, and since that time my natural state of being had become progressively more relaxed and focused. I could now be "in the zone" on a more regular basis.

I owed this change to my consistent practice of Open-Focus Attention, which has been scientifically proven to improve brain function. It is helpful to understand the science behind Open Focus, but practicing it is the best way to appreciate its real value.

I share this advice with my clients, who report improvements in their ability to remain relaxed and focused as soon as they begin practicing Open Focus.

The History of Open Focus

What is neurofeedback and how does it work? Neurofeedback involves using technology to record brainwave activity. It also helps people train their brains to maintain more relaxed and coherent brainwave activity. Dr. Les Fehmi is a neurofeedback expert out of Princeton, New Jersey, who discovered Open Focus and wrote the book, along with his colleague Jim Robbins.

At the start of his research, Dr. Fehmi discovered that no matter how many hours he spent with his biofeedback equipment, he was unable to produce the desired alpha waves (indicating a relaxed brain). When he finally stopped trying, while still attached to the biofeedback equipment, the alpha waves showed up naturally.

It took Dr. Fehmi time and effort to formulate what he had observed into two simple but profound discoveries. The first was that Narrow-Focus Attention (i.e., "zooming in") creates incoherent brainwave activity associated with stress and anxiety.

The second was that Open-Focus Attention (i.e., "zooming out"), focusing on the periphery and a point of interest at the same time, creates brain coherence and optimal performance. Essentially, this is the relaxed but focused state we know as being "in the zone."

Dr. Fehmi created a series of Open-Focus exercises to train the brain to focus this way. The exercises cover a number of specific areas (anxiety, pain, sports, etc.), but they all have one thing in common: guiding the participant to imagine the **space** around a particular object of attention.

"I Need Space" Really Means "I Need ME"

Now, let's remember our earlier discussion. We are more energy and space than physical matter. Recognizing this led me to a profound realization: the expression "I need space" really means "I need *me.*"

Furthermore, "I need space" means "I am too caught up in my emotions, and I need to get back in touch with ME so that I can figure out how to improve this situation."

We have all experienced having to give ourselves space, but we usually wait until the stress becomes unbearable. Only then do we take a step back and allow our minds to clear. **Since space is the greater part of our identity, can you think of any reason that paying attention to it should not be our highest priority?**

It is helpful to think of Narrow-Focus Attention as "doing" and Open-Focus Attention as "being." We need them both, but they need to be in balance. This is especially true when it comes to managing our emotions. The moment we zoom in and try to control our emotions, the intensity only increases. Clearly the time has come to add some "being" (space, energy) to our "doing."

Here is an example of the power of Open Focus and how it can inspire us to be our best.

Erin's Open-Focus Experience

Last year, Erin, an 18-year-old girl with a long history of treatment-resistant depression, was referred to me. We discussed a number of topics (also discussed in this book), including the importance of Open-Focus Attention.

The next day she still appeared depressed, but she claimed to feel better and said that Open Focus was starting to make sense to her. She also casually added, "I called my friend who I had been fighting with and apologized to her, and she apologized to me, and today we are meeting for lunch."

Awesome, right?

I didn't tell her to do this. I didn't even know she had a conflict with her friend. Before practicing Open Focus, she was zoomed in on "the problem," the drama of "I am right and she is wrong." When she opened her focus she created more brain coherence, gained access to her own wisdom, and took action accordingly.

That is the power of Open Focus and an example of what you can experience for yourself when you make focusing this way a priority in your life.

Keeping It Simple: Focus on the Sky to Cope with the Clouds

What does it mean in practical terms to focus on the sky to cope with the clouds? One of my favorite analogies is to think of a big open sky as the greater part of our identity. The "clouds" represent the content in our lives, including our thoughts, emotions, and of course, clinical rotations.

I'll ask you the same question that I ask my clients. "When you get some clouds in your 'sky,' do you focus on the open sky and the clouds or do you just zoom in on the clouds?"

Like most people I have asked, I bet you are sheepishly shaking your head and thinking, I just zoom in on the clouds, even though I know I should be looking at the sky (the big picture).

Don't feel bad. This is something our culture has trained us to do. But now we have to change all this and retrain our brains into learning the skill of Open-Focus Attention. So let's move on to the introductory exercise that I share with my clients.

Open Focus: An Introductory Exercise

Imagine the space in the room where you are sitting as the greater part of you. Crumple a piece of paper into a ball (representing a cloud), place it on a table, and sit comfortably in a chair. Focus on the cloud in two different ways, and take notice of how you feel in your brain and body as you shift your attention.

First, zoom in on the cloud and try to block out everything else, as if you were a camera focusing a close-up shot. Then, slowly start zooming out to include other things into your awareness but don't take your eyes off the cloud (the paper ball).

I don't expect you to see the complete shape of each object in the periphery but simply to notice that they are there. Also, don't try to label everything, just be aware that other objects exist in that space in addition to the cloud.

When I am working with clients, I ask them the following types of questions: Can you see some of the window to the right? How about a bit of the carpet? Can you see the chair to your left? As you are opening your focus, how are you feeling in your body?

I then ask them to zoom in and out a few times on their own and report how they are feeling.

Typical responses include:

"I feel like I can't breathe when I zoom in and more relaxed when I zoom out."

"I feel constricted when zoomed in and open when I zoom out."

"Oh my God, I totally see what you mean!"

Go ahead and try this, and notice how you feel as you zoom in and zoom out on your own. I would be surprised if you did not notice a profound difference.

After taking clients through this exercise, I remind them that when we focus on the clouds, we get more clouds. But when we focus on the sky, we gain access to infinite possibilities that we cannot see when we have such tunnel vision.

Open-Focus Attention: The Key to a Peaceful, Successful Life

Open-Focus Attention is the foundation for health and optimal performance. This is how we are focused when we are in the zone. So doesn't it make sense to make this focus a priority? A commitment to the practice of Open-Focus Attention would surely improve your chances of having a successful clinical rotation.

However, as you will likely discover, staying in Open Focus is not always easy because we have been conditioned to focus in a very narrow, fixated way. Open Focus feels unnatural initially, but it does get easier with practice.

Here is another story illustrating the importance of Open Focus and how forgetting to practice can be detrimental to our well-being.

"Success" without Peace Is NOT Success

I was recently working with a woman who had made a serious suicide attempt. She was very successful in her career, having been with the same organization for 35 years.

I took her through a brief Open Focus exercise, and she did not like it at all. Why? She had created a great deal of external success using extreme Narrow-Focus Attention. In fact, she communicated this, saying, "It works for me."

I smiled as I replied, "I don't like to get Dr. Phil on people, but how is it *really* working for you?"

I know this woman's experience (attempted suicide) is quite extreme but there is a tremendous imbalance between "doing" and "being" in our culture. Many people live in an almost constant state of stress for this reason.

This problem needs to be addressed, and practicing Open Focus is the answer. Open Focus is a powerful training tool that teaches you how to be relaxed and focused (goal oriented) at the same time—a key component to your success.

Open-Focus Attention: The KEY to "Upgrading Your Software"

Even though we are perfect at our core, we are all plagued with imperfect human conditioning. Identifying with our conditioning is one of our most destructive habits.

Here are a few examples of this self-identification.

"I **am** a worrier" as opposed to "I worry sometimes."

"I **am** angry" as opposed to "I get angry sometimes."

"I **am** a loser" as opposed to "I lose sometimes."

The list goes on and on, but I am certain you get the idea.

As long as I believe "I **am** a worrier," there is no possible way I can change. The truth is that I am much more the **space** around the worry than the worry itself. This is not opinion, it is absolute fact, and here is where the power of Open-Focus Attention comes into play.

Practicing Open Focus, literally being the space around life's clouds, can break the identification with destructive conditioning. By zooming out and not giving the clouds *all* of our attention, we literally free up energy and gain access to a greater intelligence—our intuition. This enables us to make more empowering and empowered choices.

Open Focus is a very simple skill to learn, but our conditioning runs deep. We have layers and layers of outdated "software" and "viruses" (junk) that make it more difficult to remain in our natural Open-Focus state.

Now that you have a basic understanding of the Human Operating System, we will discuss how we can change the conditioning that prevents regular access to our most natural state of being. The following chapters will expand your knowledge and help you remain in an Open-Focus state.

LOOKING IN THE MIRROR

Turning Down the Anxiety Volume

I recently worked with George, a very anxious young man, who could barely sit still and make eye contact. He'd been on the unit for a couple of weeks. While he was generally cooperative, he was easily frustrated by other people and had difficulty being around them.

During the course of our session, I noticed a dramatic shift in the level of George's anxiety, which, he told me, decreased from a 10 to a 5. A number of ideas that I put forward seemed to resonate with him. The concept of Open-Focus Attention was most helpful.

My colleagues (who worked with him on the unit) reported several positive behavioral changes the next day, including an increased ability to tolerate being around people, and the fact that he seemed less anxious.

One of my colleagues reported that a number of things helped create this dramatic shift in George's behavior. I wanted to ask George directly if he could specify what he found most helpful.

The more conscious he is about what is really working for him, the more likely he can repeat the behavior in the future. Also, I like to get feedback so that I know what treatments are most effective.

When I asked George, without any hesitation, and even with a little excitement, he started telling me how practicing Open Focus was making a "night and day" difference.

He was able to articulate *how* it was working for him, stating, "I'm not just zooming in on the anxiety cloud, so I am able to relax more and question where it might be coming from, instead of automatically going into panic mode." In other words, George was *empowered* by knowing exactly how to manage his anxiety.

KEY #3: THE SCIENCE OF EMOTION

Emotions = Energy in Motion

Think of the brain and body as an energetic hose. Consider what happens when you "kink" the brain by fixating on emotional clouds. The flow of energy slows down and pressure starts building up, and this is NOT just a psychological buildup.

The word *emotion* translates to "energy in motion." Excessive Narrow Focus disrupts the normal flow of energy that keeps us healthy and working efficiently. It drains our energy resources and creates the feeling of having low energy or being "stuck."

Understanding the science of emotion will help you keep your energy up—a key component to your success.

Emotions Are Chemicals

The documentary *What the Bleep Do We Know* beautifully illustrates the chemical nature of emotion. We tend to think of emotions as something abstract or psychological. But there is a specific chemical blend that matches every emotion we experience.

Emotions are also extremely addictive, chemically binding to the same cell receptor sites in the brain as heroin does for a user (Pert, *Molecules of Emotion*). Consider what this means.

It means that, like a heroin addict, we feel extremely uncomfortable without our fix, which may be a mix of chemicals that create worry, anger, self-sabotage, the need to please, etc.

These states of being do not feel good but they are at least familiar, and they give us a sense of identity (e.g., "I am a worrier"). Change is difficult because, like alcoholics who stop drinking, we will go through withdrawal.

In other words, we have to feel different than usual, a state that causes the body to rebel the moment change is attempted (Dispenza, *Breaking the Habit*). For example, you may have a powerful urge to lie on the couch instead of going to the gym. The moment you give in to the urge, you reinforce the "I am lazy" identity. Don't beat yourself up about it, though; that will just reinforce another layer of conditioning.

The key is to be aware of when this is happening so that you can intervene and make a conscious choice before your body automatically takes control.

What does this have to do with clinical success?

Remember, **attention to the present moment is the *key* to optimal performance.** We often lose the present moment by unconsciously reacting in ways such as

—trying to control negative thoughts, like "I don't know what I'm doing!"

—trying to impress a supervisor.

—being too concerned about results.

—feeling overwhelmed/not able to manage the caseload.

—just wanting to be done.

—being distracted by social media.

—having difficulty managing work/life balance.

If you are not fully aware and paying attention, you can easily "get lost" and limit your ability to access your greatest intelligence. You do not want this to happen during your clinical rotations.

Emotional Awareness: The Key to Your Greatest Intelligence

Emotional Awareness is the backdrop to the popular concept of Emotional Intelligence, since it is **awareness** that enables us to be intelligent about our emotions. Awareness is a state of **knowing**; it has little to do with thinking or analysis.

The story about the young woman who apologized to her friend is a good example. She did not think about or analyze her decision, it happened automatically. This was only possible because she first became more emotionally aware, which naturally resulted in her choosing an emotionally intelligent action.

Unconscious thinking and behavior create the majority of our problems, which is why history tends to repeat itself. Emotional Awareness makes it possible to "change history" by rising above our conditioned habits and to think in innovative, emotionally intelligent ways that produce optimal results.

Emotional Awareness is not about learning new information. It is about tuning in to your intuition. Deep down, you already know everything you need to know about Emotional Awareness. However, the following six reminders and accompanying diagrams will help you tap into your wisdom more consistently.

1. You Are Awareness

Do you ever find yourself caught up in the drama between the "angel" (higher self) and the "devil" (lower self) as they jockey for position? This is the "I should work out, but I don't want to, but I really should" phenomenon.

The "Voice" In Your Head is Not You!
It's just the Silly Little Ego

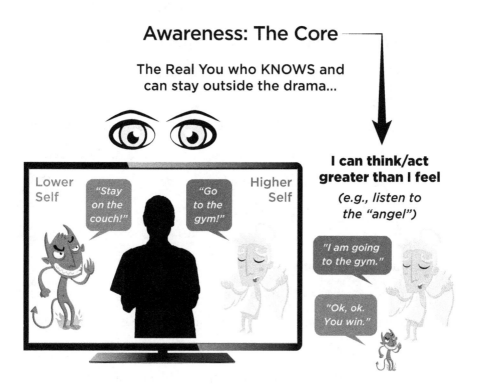

Remember, you are *not* the angel or devil. You are the Awareness that *knows* they exist.

People complain about being too stressed but they like (are used to) the drama created by this kind of internal dialogue. Suppose I am trying to reduce my sugar intake but am used to eating ice cream every night. My internal dialogue would sound something like this:

"I so badly want some ice cream! It's really not that bad for me, and I'm not overweight, so it's totally fine. But my cholesterol is high, so I really shouldn't. I don't know what to do. Yes, I do; I'm not going to have it, but this is so hard!"

We underestimate the emotional toll this type of inner dialogue has on our well-being. We create our own struggle, but it does not have to be this way.

Habits are easier to break once we start living from our core. The reason is that we can observe the angel and devil without getting caught in the middle, effectively staying *outside* the drama. Only then can we follow the wise advice of the angel.

2. Stay outside the Drama

Once I am operating from Awareness (the real me), I can **observe** the push and pull of the angel and devil and make a conscious choice NOT to have the ice cream.

I might still have the craving, but I am less likely to act on it because **I am *outside* of the urge**. This enables me to think and choose wisely, bypassing the drama. It's that simple.

Staying present and breaking unhealthy habits is ultimately more satisfying than indulging in a momentary treat, but we must also remember the importance of intention. Our actions do not matter nearly as much as the intention behind them.

3. Remain Aware of Your Intention

It took me several years to notice that I was accessing the zone to help others, not just to be myself. Although I remained relatively peaceful, I did feel tension at times from worrying about results. ("Am I helping?") After a session I would immediately go back "home" (in my head) and impatiently look for my next fix.

It was *exhausting*.

I believe this is a relatively common issue among healthcare professionals. I know many who cannot allow for themselves the compassionate, caring attention that they provide to their patients. It is easy to fall into this trap when we forget who we are behind the roles we play.

4. You Are NOT the Roles You Play

You will play many roles in your life, but none of them are the real YOU. I know this is a tough pill to swallow, especially because the ego loves to disguise itself as a serious healthcare professional. It had me fooled for years before I got in touch with the real me behind my role as a therapist. The way we unconsciously identify with our roles can be very subtle but worth exploring.

Trust me, you do not want to make the mistake of confusing **what you do** with **who you are**. It creates a great deal of pressure to be perfect ("I *should* know!") and reinforces the feeling of separation between the patient and provider. We should indeed take our role(s) seriously, just not ourselves (Karl Ardo, Mentor). Understanding and practicing this will make the roles you play more enjoyable and fulfilling.

5. Being Aware (Present) Is the Ultimate Satisfaction

I have finally learned that being present is the only thing (it's not really a "thing") that offers long-term satisfaction (Tolle, *A New Earth*). Everything external, like helping others, a great meal, vacation, or new car, is fleeting. No matter how wonderful the particular pleasure may be, we can never be fully satisfied until we are aware of our connection to something greater. All that is required to feel that connection is attention to the present moment.

I know this all sounds so incredibly simple, but putting it into practice is not always easy. The reason is that we are conditioned to run away from the present moment, unconsciously trying to find ourselves in the external world. But research shows that we can train (rewire the brain) ourselves to live in the present—it is our natural state. It boils down to staying conscious, outside of old reactive patterns, one moment at a time.

6. You CAN Rewire Your Brain

Think of the frontal lobe as the executive decision maker. Its job is to help the body stay focused while guiding it to perform healthy behaviors. Your job is to ensure that it is performing its function properly. Remember, **you** (the human operator) are the boss, and the frontal lobe is your subordinate.

The problem is that we human operators are not very good at paying attention. We often let our subordinate (the brain and body) call the shots, and it chooses short-term gratification over long-term fulfillment.

The key to regaining control is to start **paying attention to *how* and *where* our attention is placed.**

First, we need to consider the object of our attention: Is it positive or negative? Second, are we in Open Focus or Narrow Focus?

We have all had the experience of feeling great one moment and horrible the next. When this occurs, the brain is actually changing from coherent to incoherent activity. Dr. Fannin defines this as a "phase shift."

I asked Dr. Fannin if that is why you can feel lousy one second and great the next after running into a friendly golden retriever.

"Exactly," he replied.

Most people think it cannot be that easy to break free of a bad mood, but it really is simple. Sustaining the improved mood requires repetition, but at any moment a simple shift *can* and *will* initiate positive momentum.

If it is that simple, then why do we not practice it?

Narrow-Focus Attention has become our default mode, especially when it comes to our emotions. Instead of staying open, many of us fixate and try to control our emotional clouds. Others react externally and project them onto something outside of themselves (like road rage).

Either of these reactions can instantly transform a peaceful person into a road rager. These reactions also reinforce the brain's and body's reactive patterns and the familiar feelings (stress, anger, etc.), keeping us unconscious and inside the box.

When we simply **observe** our emotions in Open Focus we can remain conscious, outside of the old reactive behaviors. This practice can help prevent automatic reactions, and it becomes easier to stop

Awareness:
"The Human Operator"

Rewiring New Programs of Behavior

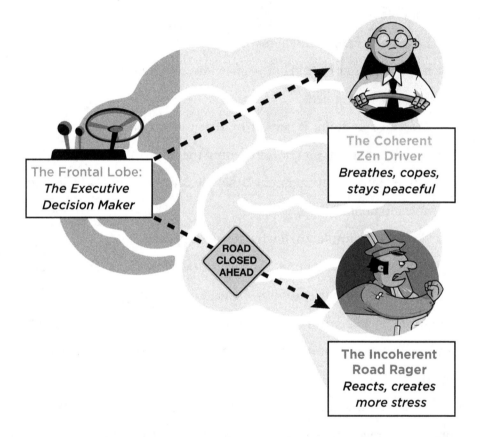

The Frontal Lobe:
The Executive Decision Maker

The Coherent Zen Driver
Breathes, copes, stays peaceful

ROAD CLOSED AHEAD

The Incoherent Road Rager
Reacts, creates more stress

the program that is running wild. This practice will also make it progressively more natural for you to live in the zone.

It does, however, take effort. Imagine training a five-year-old dog that has never been disciplined. Do you think he will follow your commands? Will he fight you to stay in control?

Guess what "animal" behaves the same way?

Your body, of course. But you *can* learn to be its master (Dispenza). The training and rewiring starts by teaching your body to *sit*, *stay*, and *heel*, meaning **to stay present**, as you manage your never-ending to-do list.

Manage Your To-Do List, Don't Let It Manage You!

I ask clients, "How do you feel when looking at all the items on your to-do list?" Typical responses include "I feel really stressed out"; "I feel really overwhelmed"; and "I don't even want to think about it."

How do you feel when you think about everything you have to do to graduate?

Most of us immediately become stressed the moment we think about our list, and here is why. We instantaneously **react** (without knowing it) to the first "hit" (e.g., "How am I ever going to get all this done?!"), turning it into an explosion that leads to **stress.**

We start mentally and physically bouncing through our lists, which attracts chemicals of fear, frustration, anxiety, and doubt. We are not stressed because of our to-dos but because we are *thinking* about the entire list all at the same time.

No one likes to feel stressed, so what do we do?

We run!

Many of us go into overdrive trying to get everything done (usually an impossible task), while unconsciously self-medicating with junk food, social media, alcohol, TV, you name it. Interrupting the natural flow of energy in this way can take the body out of its homeostasis, potentially leading to mental and physical disease.

All we have to do to remain healthy, balanced, and productive is to make "catching ourselves" and coming back to the present moment our highest priority. This is not just psychologically healthy, but it may be the healthiest natural medicine on the planet.

Consider how you feel when you get something off your chest or shift from being overwhelmed to being relaxed but focused.

The common response is "I feel relieved," and for good reason. We interrupted the flow of negativity, released energy, and guided ourselves back to the present moment. No wonder it feels great.

But back to dog training and managing our to-do lists.

Dogs may sit only for a moment after they first learn the command "Sit." The dog is going to try to run because the command is not yet fully programmed into his brain. The human body is the same way. We must initially keep it (like the dog) on a very short leash.

I can now give my "dog" a longer leash than in the past, but I still must watch him closely. It does take effort, but the reward, just being myself, is immeasurable.

The Two Benefits of "Staying" (Being Present)

Learning to "stay" has two primary benefits: we feel better, and we become more productive. You must meet the same criteria to graduate, regardless of how you feel inside. Can you think of any reason why staying present should not be your highest priority?

Give up the delusion that you are going to feel that much better when you graduate. It will feel amazing, but I assure you, the feeling will not last very long.

Unless you are aware of your connection to something greater (yourself), you will soon be racing toward the next future moment (advancement, $, marriage, kids, etc.), missing out on the only thing that ever matters: right now.

The worst part of our destructive habits is that we cannot fully appreciate our successes. As Alan Watts stated, "What is the point of planning for a future that you will not be there to enjoy?"

Start training your "puppy" to sit, stay, and heel **now**, so you will fully enjoy all the fruits of your labor.

LOOKING IN THE MIRROR

Staying Present: One Moment at a Time

Ten years ago, I had a profound aha! moment that changed my life. I was just beginning to learn the basics of "The Formula" after being emotionally stuck for a very long time. I had a 10-year to-do list that I wanted to complete but had not even started.

I went to Target to get picture frames because that was the first item on my list. In the midst of frantically racing around the store, I became **aware** (of a surge of chemicals), stopped, and consciously thought, I am feeling overwhelmed because I am thinking about my entire list. This isn't just psychological; I am actually creating more chemicals of stress by thinking this way. All I came here to do today was get picture frames. I don't need to think about anything else.

I felt a palpable sense of release, and I gained a deeper understanding of the chemical nature of emotions (that just flooded my brain), and how I could positively influence my mood simply by paying attention.

I could not explain it this way at the time, but it was my first conscious experience of focusing on the "sky" while noticing the "clouds." My "inner dog" was starting to learn and that was because I was finally doing my job of being its master.

I share this example since many students go into overdrive when feeling overwhelmed, especially with the demands of their clinical rotations. This creates a great imbalance and the buildup of stress, which can lead to performance issues and even physical illness.

The value of simply paying attention and "catching" yourself is immeasurable. It is the foundation for programming yourself to be calm and focused.

I share the following with clients: "I catch myself hundreds of times a day. It does take effort, but it is totally worth it. I'm gaining energy each time I catch myself and return to the present moment, instead of draining my energy by working in overdrive."

CHAPTER 3

THE BASIC FORMULA

It is now time to take your "inner puppy" to obedience class. You may be saying, "I don't need to, this is so simple, I already got this." It is simple, but do not be fooled. The strategies we use to trick ourselves into thinking "I get it" when we don't are extremely complex. I would be a millionaire if I had a nickel for every time I thought I got it, only to find myself falling into the same familiar traps.

As my boss, Lila, said, "If you cannot consistently demonstrate something in your life, then you don't know it."

This is *not* about learning new information. It is about gaining wisdom, and that can only be acquired through experience.

What good is it to know "I shouldn't worry" if you cannot stop yourself from worrying? I am inviting you to lay down your "I already know this" voice as you work through this book. It will help you "get it" in a deeper, more meaningful way.

As Dr. Joe Dispenza teaches, it is not enough to do it one, ten, or even a hundred times; we must practice until the body knows better than the mind—until it becomes a habit. Staying present can and will become your new habit. All it takes is a little of your attention and energy. The rest of the formula is about getting to know the real you and rising above conditioning that sometimes gets in your way.

Although we will expand on this, just collecting more information is not going to do the trick. You must apply what you are learning to achieve the ultimate reward—**wisdom.**

I think of human beings as shaken-up soda bottles. We have a lot of pressure built up inside. Applying what you learn in this book has two primary benefits that will help you deal with the pressure. First, it will prevent you from building up more pressure; second, it will show you how to relieve pressure by "slowly untwisting the cap" in a way that feels right for you.

However, before you go any further, remember.

There is NOTHING wrong with YOU. YOU are perfect at your CORE.

This is not just some Pollyanna remark; it is an absolute truth. We are not our behaviors. The process of change becomes much easier when we stop beating ourselves up ("I'm a loser!") for our human conditioning.

For example, "I am such a jerk for letting people take advantage of me" becomes "It is not healthy to let people take advantage of me. I want to learn how to become more assertive."

When we stop taking our conditioning so personally, we naturally become more joyful and inspired, and change becomes easier. So let's review.

KEY POINTS

1. You are the awareness that **knows** (not the thinker).
2. You are mostly made of space/energy.
3. You are perfect at your core.
4. Open Focus is the key to staying in the zone.

5. You are the master who can train your body to "stay."

6. Emotional Awareness is the key to your greatest intelligence.

7. Being present is the greatest reward.

8. Learning to "stay" is a moment-by-moment process.

The Formula

The book *A Course in Miracles* teaches that the reason you are upset is never the real reason, because you will never run out of reasons for being upset.

The real reason is that we have lost ourselves in the external world. I am not suggesting that we should never be upset about anything. I am referring to the many instances in which we become overly upset and reactive.

The formula for getting back on track is always the same, regardless of the trigger (school, money, relationships, illness, etc.). It boils down to paying attention, staying aware, and choosing healthy responses, instead of going on emotional autopilot.

Remembering the following guidelines keeps you focused. When in doubt, just think about "The Formula" and follow the sequence.

The General Formula

The General Formula consists of three basic principles that are the foundation for staying present. They are simple on the surface but deeply powerful when put into practice.

<u>STEP 1</u>: Acceptance is the biggest reliever of stress. **Be honest with yourself.**

- Accept things as they are, not as they should be (Chopra).
- Global acceptance: "Yes, I don't like it, but I have a ton of work to do before graduation."
- Moment: "I really don't want to do this assignment right now, but I must do it anyway."
- There are levels of acceptance: "How would I feel if I truly accepted this?" It would be a nonissue. If it is still an issue, then it is not fully accepted.
- Acceptance can be a process that happens over time.

STEP 2: Take Responsibility: "I am 100% responsible for my own emotional state."

- Complaining/Blaming = Giving away power by allowing an external factor to control your internal state.
- Taking responsibility = Keeping your power by doing whatever is necessary to maintain a healthy emotional state.

STEP 3: Commitment: Constant and never-ending improvement (W. Edwards Deming).

- We never reach the finish line; there is always room for improvement.

The Moment-by-Moment Formula

The Moment-by-Moment Formula was created to help stay on track when you are triggered emotionally. When things are running smoothly, we often naturally go through these steps unconsciously—it just happens. But we can quickly lose that ability when we are triggered emotionally.

By learning to slow down and pause (like watching a DVD frame by frame), we can consciously use the formula to our advantage.

Step 1. Feel/Be Aware/Embrace when something "hits" you.

Step 2. Pause and "Create your Space" (Viktor Frankl).

Step 3. Understand. "What exactly am I feeling? What is the situation?"

Step 4. Choose Response and let go of Outcome.

Step 5. Learn. "What did I do well? Where did I fall off track? How can I do better next time?"

Step 6. Validate, validate, validate. Subtle shifts in thinking = **huge** changes in reality. Patting ourselves on the back is an essential life skill.

Staying Connected: The Top 3 Tools

Nothing is more important than staying connected to your core (awareness). It will make everything you do in your life significantly easier and more enjoyable. The following exercises are three simple ways to make staying connected a natural part of your life. I recommend practicing them as often as possible; they are very powerful.

TOOL #1: THE MOST IMPORTANT THINGS
—LIST AND REVIEW

My all-time favorite quote is, "The most important thing is to remember the most important thing" (unknown origin).

Would you agree that being at peace (just being yourself) is the most important thing? How often do you think about that? I have asked many people this question, and the frequent response is, "Almost never."

Many of us forget about what is most important as we pursue external things (degrees, money, recognition, etc.) that give only momentary satisfaction. Writing down and reviewing what is most important to you is one of the easiest and most effective tools for maintaining focus. How could you possibly not perform at your best if you are always focusing on what is most important to you?

I recommend creating a list of the **Three Most Important Things** that remind you of your deepest intentions.

Here is my current list:

1. Sense the space/energy in and around my body.

2. Joy is my highest priority.

3. Do the best I can in whatever I am doing.

Do I remember these all the time? No, but since I remind myself of them as often as possible, I am usually quite peaceful and productive. My tendency to spiral into negativity has significantly declined since making this exercise a regular part of my practice.

My "down days" are directly related to forgetting to review my Three Most Important Things. You can experiment and see what feels right to you. Feel free to modify your list as you continue to grow and evolve.

TOOL #2: "FEELING I"

The greater part of who we are is Energy. Paying attention to the energy field in the body is a simple way to stay connected to the real you (Tolle). It is also an easy way to reduce your stress-producing internal dialogue.

Here is what you do: Close your eyes and feel the energy in your hands. It might be helpful to ask yourself, "How can I know my hands are there without looking at them?" You will notice that you can feel them. Once connected, repeat the following statement (internally or externally) for three minutes: "I am this feeling, this feeling is me . . . I am this feeling . . . this feeling is me."

"Feeling I" will immediately bring you into a state of peace. It will also establish a new connection in your brain—"I am Energy." In other words, you will break your identification with the mental story of your life that causes unnecessary stress.

Yesterday, I ran into a client I worked with nearly three years ago. He said, "I was feeling really stressed the other day, and I did that hand thing. It made me feel more balanced right away." I am so inspired (to practice and teach) when I hear about people using these tools to improve the quality of their lives.

TOOL #3: CONSCIOUS MOVEMENT

"It is the journey that matters, not so much the destination." We **know** this but often forget while racing toward the future. This causes us to miss out on the amazing gifts that are available by simply paying attention to our senses.

Before reading on, go ahead and take a 30-second walk around the room you're in right now.

AFTER YOUR BRIEF WALK

Ask yourself, "What did I notice?" You are probably saying, "Not very much," and this is because we are simply not conditioned to pay attention.

Now, go ahead and take the same walk again, only this time pay attention and see what you can pick up on with your senses. There is no right or wrong way to do this little exercise.

AFTER YOUR CONSCIOUS BRIEF WALK

Now, ask yourself, "What did I notice? What did I see? What did I hear? Did I feel anything? Did I smell anything? How am I feeling *right now*? How did the first walk compare to the second?"

You may find yourself being noticeably more relaxed. This is because you took your attention away from the analytical mind by paying attention to your senses. Imagine how you would feel if you did that as often as possible throughout your day. Conscious movement is an easy, alternative way to practice Open-Focus Attention.

A few months ago, I introduced a client to these tools. He looked considerably better the next day. When I asked him if he'd been practicing, he said, "Yes, I took that conscious walk. I see what you mean—it really works." He continued practicing and left our unit looking so much better than when he was admitted.

Preparing for Optimal Performance

Now that you are familiar with the Human Operating System and The Formula, it is time to deepen your understanding by exploring related topics and practicing recommended exercises. The following chapters are designed to help you prepare yourself for optimal performance. They include:

- **Scanning for "Viruses"** (Identifying Negative Traits and Beliefs)

- **Upgrading Your Software** (Programming Positive Thoughts and Beliefs)
- **Rebooting Your System** (Understanding the Power of Acceptance)
- **"Clearing Cookies"** (Using Energy to Stay "In the Zone")
- **Keeping Your System Updated** (Creating Your Plan of Action)
- **Troubleshooting** (Diagnosing and Treating Challenges)

Exploring these chapters will make it progressively easier to stay present. It will also teach you many shortcuts for "coming home" when you get off track.

The Basic Formula: Recommended/Related Resources

Ultimately, we must each explore whatever resources feel right to us. While there are thousands of great resources out there, in my experience only a select few really cut to the chase. Here is a list of some that I consider essential and most relevant to our current discussion.

1. *A New Earth* (Tolle)
2. *Breaking the Habit of Being Yourself* (Dispenza)
3. *The Open-Focus Brain* (Fehmi/Robbins)
4. *The Power of Now* (Tolle)
5. *You Are the Placebo* (Dispenza)
6. *What the Bleep Do We Know* (DVD)

The Formula Always Works

One of my colleagues is more of a natural at staying present. She doesn't sweat the small stuff and is a "Jedi Master" at working with children.

She took an interest in what I was teaching because it scientifically explained what she was already doing. She didn't have the words or "Formula" that outlined how or why it worked—for her, it just happened automatically. This may sound strange: she was more aware, yet she wasn't aware of this particular fact.

Why does it matter?

No matter where we are in life, there is always room to improve our "game." The more we understand the *why* and *how*, the better the Formula works and the more we can use it to our advantage.

My colleague has been married for over 30 years. She and her husband have a great relationship but they do have their issues—one of them involves cooking and cleaning. She cooks, and he is supposed to wash the dishes. Until fairly recently, it was always a battle to get him to do his job. Everything changed when she became more AWARE of her role in the conflict.

One day she told me, "You're not going to believe this. Last night, I decided I wasn't going to say anything to him about the dishes. After we ate, I felt the urge to nudge him, but instead, I just went up to my room to read. This morning, I came downstairs to find that not only had he washed the dishes, he cleaned the entire kitchen!"

This happened a few years ago. When I recently told her that I wanted to include the story in this book, she laughed as she said, "My husband just told one of our friends that I don't like having dirty dishes left in the sink." It seems like the new behavior (washing the dishes) has stuck and the Formula worked.

CHAPTER 4

SCANNING FOR "VIRUSES"

The human brain is the world's most sophisticated computer. As such, it does not always work at full capacity since it can also be inflicted with "viruses." These viruses operate like unconscious programs, sabotaging our efforts through an endless supply of negative thoughts, feelings, and beliefs. They can slow us down and even make us crash.

We live in such a "just think positive" culture. It's a great idea in theory, but it doesn't always work, and here is why. Many of us skip the first and most essential step of understanding why we feel bad in the first place. It is nearly impossible to think positive without first acknowledging and accepting what we are feeling.

Author Debbie Ford once said, "You can put ice cream on top of poop, but you are still going to taste the poop." It is a gross analogy but accurate. We do not want to dwell on the negative, but we do need to "own" its existence.

Research has shown that an emotion will pass in about 90 seconds when we allow the energy to flow naturally. But **the immune system takes eight hours to recover from just a five-minute emotional reaction** (Dispenza, *You Are the Placebo*).

Turning on Your Light

Deepak Chopra said, "You cannot fight darkness with darkness, but you can turn on the light." Imagine having a basement full of junk. It would be nearly impossible to clean it without first turning on the light. Seeing what is there can be a little scary and overwhelming, but it is an essential part of the process. The same is true for our dark thoughts, feelings, and qualities that we try to hide.

The documentary *The Shadow Effect* illustrates that we all have the capacity to embody and express every quality in existence. We can be loving but also hateful, compassionate but also judgmental, etc.

Many of us were taught to deny our negative qualities, which leads to what Debbie Ford calls the Beach-Ball Effect. When we try to hold a beach ball underwater, it pops right up! The same is true for any personality trait or emotion that we try to hide.

Here is a personal example. A few years ago, my golf buddy said, "Dan, you seem like such a calm guy, so I am always surprised to see you get so angry when playing golf."

At that time, I had not yet learned that by denying my tendency to get angry, I was limiting my ability to choose to remain calm. Instead, I was exploding. Once I started "scanning for viruses," my ability to remain calm dramatically increased. I still get angry, but I rarely explode because I stopped denying this part of my true nature.

Looking for viruses (negative traits) appears counterintuitive in our "just think positive" culture, but it is necessary. It takes a great deal of energy to block out qualities that make us human.

Initially, this can be uncomfortable, and you may notice your silly little ego saying, "This is a waste of time; I don't want to do this." But that is just a defense mechanism, or your body's attempt to maintain its "safe," familiar state of being.

The value of spending a little bit of time scanning for viruses is immeasurable. Once the "basement" has been cleared out, we are left with empty space and more power to choose the very qualities we would like to emulate on a regular basis.

KEY POINTS

1. We all embody every quality that exists.
2. Denying any quality ("I'm NOT that!") limits our ability to choose.
3. The world is our mirror. (We judge people who remind us of ourselves.)
4. "I can be angry sometimes" does *not* equal "I AM ANGRY!"
5. Scanning for viruses is an **empowering** action.
6. Scanning for viruses literally frees up energy.

Scanning for Viruses: The Best Tool to Get Started

Scanning for viruses is a process that never ends. No matter how much internal work we have done, there is always room for more exploration. And just like with real computers, new viruses are constantly being created, so we must keep our anti-viral software up to date.

Remember, we are **not** our emotions. Even if an old man has been angry for 60 years, anger is **not** his identity; it is **not** his real self. The exercise below, adapted from Debbie Ford's book *The Dark Side of Light*

Chasers, is essential to breaking the identification with our emotions—the root cause of suffering.

Create a chart and list as many of your qualities that come to mind. I encourage you to devote some time to self-reflection. The qualities of which we deny ownership are often *very* good at hiding and will not be apparent at first. I assure you, the benefit of this exercise is well worth the effort.

The chart should include both negative qualities or "Non-Ideal," and positive or "Ideal" qualities. I recommend starting with the negatives. Be sure to include the ones that really hurt to admit. They are your biggest energy drainers. Then, complete the positive side. We often tend to deny our greatness, which keeps us in the safe but mediocre zone.

I find it easier to organize this exercise in alphabetical order; i.e., identifying as many qualities as you can that begin with each letter (A for angry, arrogant; B for bad, blamer; C for cold, careless, etc.). Below is an example of how you might get started.

Pay attention to how you feel as you are creating your list. It may hurt on some level, like, "Yes, this is true, but I don't want to admit it." Remember that you are not discovering anything new. You are becoming conscious of what may be limiting your potential. It can be unsettling at first, but that feeling won't last for long. Most people report feeling lighter for being honest.

"Non-Ideal" Qualities I can sometimes be...	"Ideal" Qualities But, I can also be...
A. angry, agitated, annoyed	A. aware, awesome, alive
B. bad, belligerent, bullying	B. beautiful, bold, brave

Scanning for Viruses: Recommended/Related Resources

1. *Daring Greatly* (Brown)
2. *The Dark Side of Light Chasers* (Ford)
3. "Listening to Shame" (TED Talks; Brené Brown)
4. "The Power of Vulnerability" (TED Talks; Brené Brown)
5. *The Shadow Effect* (DVD)

The World IS Our Mirror

While this might sound ironic, the attending physician who used to run one of our units was clearly mentally troubled. She could be extremely rude and downright nasty to the patients on the unit, which left many of them in an awkward position. The majority of them were scared (rightly so) to speak their mind or complain, in fear of retribution.

Nadine, a very guarded, tough-looking woman was referred to me. We really connected, and it wasn't long before I started hearing about how she was butting heads with the physician. The doctor briefly pulled her out during one of our sessions. Nadine left in a great mood but returned, yelling, "God demit, she did it again!"

This led to a discussion about how the qualities we despise in others are the very ones we are denying in ourselves. I recommended watching *The Shadow Effect*. She did and it changed her life.

Nadine (appropriately) spoke her truth the next day in front of the treatment team, which included the doctor, nurse, social worker, and medical students (unfortunately I wasn't there to see it).

She said to her doctor, "You're my mirror and I'm your mirror. You're rude, nasty, and condescending, just like me, and that's why I don't like you."

My colleague who witnessed this said, "It was amazing. We all just sat there in silence as she said something we all knew to be true." The doctor treated her with the utmost respect from that day forward.

Even though the doctor continued to be disrespectful to other clients long after Nadine left our unit, Nadine's brutal honesty obviously impacted her. It is uncomfortable to point the finger internally in this way, but we owe it to ourselves to be honest about our least favorable traits.

CHAPTER 5

UPGRADING YOUR SOFTWARE

It is not enough to just scan for viruses; we must also eliminate them by becoming familiar with those specific thoughts and beliefs that slow us down. As we remove them, thinking positively will become natural.

Imagine having a jar full of marbles. The marbles represent negative thoughts and beliefs—viruses. The space within the jar represents the greater part of our identity, empty space, or a void of possibility. Once we clear out our own viruses, we can upgrade our software by choosing empowering "marbles" (thoughts/beliefs).

This becomes the foundation for effective communication—a key component of your clinical success. Research has shown that only 7% of communication is verbal. The main ingredient of the remaining 93% is emotion, most of which is unconscious.

Imagine trying to listen to a great song on a radio that is not tuned in properly. The song gets lost in all the static. This is what happens when we are not fully aware—we verbally and non-verbally communicate with our emotions.

Every student wants to perform their best, but they do not always communicate their intention clearly. Here are two examples of this.

Many students believe they are supposed to be perfect. As a result, they may not express their real needs, which can lead to performance issues. These students may come across as anxious, scared, and insecure.

On the flip side, other students overcompensate for their insecurity by pretending they know more than they do. They often come across as arrogant and not open to learning.

Communication issues like these are more common than you might think, and they are catalysts for many problems during clinical rotations. These issues can be easily avoided by paying closer attention to the driving force behind communication—emotion.

Stephen Covey, author of *The 7 Habits of Highly Effective People*, declares, "Seek first to understand, and then be understood." I appreciate this message, but we cannot seek to understand others without *first* understanding ourselves. The reason is that we can misinterpret others by not being aware of our own lens. It is this misinterpretation that often leads to conflict.

The key to understanding ourselves is being aware of what we are feeling in any given moment. Many of us have become so desensitized that we have no appreciation of our emotions or how they influence our communication and behavior.

A Lesson from a Dog

My friend attempted to train her dog, Jake, with a low-budget shock collar. Jake could bark twice without being shocked, but a third bark would elicit a zap. Jake learned this lesson in about 30 minutes. He started going "woof, woof," but then would open his mouth and resist the temptation to bark a third time! Jake learned that if he kept "complaining" (barking) he would only be hurting himself.

We "smart humans" underestimate the impact that negative

thinking habits have on the chemistry in our bodies. Unlike Jake, we don't always notice the shocks we give ourselves by allowing negative programs to run continually. We also expend a great deal of energy trying to numb the pain that the shocks create.

The shocks initially do hurt. This is usually because we believe they mean something negative about ourselves. The negative emotion we feel is real, but the meaning we attach to it is *not* necessarily true. Henry Ford understood this when he said, "If you think you can, or you think you can't, either way you are right."

We get to decide what we like to believe. The first step is to become familiar with what we are unconsciously accepting as true and to understand that nothing has any meaning until we decide it does.

Here is an example.

What does **"I did not get the placement I want"** mean?

Technically, it just means you didn't get the placement you wanted, but your interpretation can change the meaning very quickly. If you believe that "This is the worst thing that has happened to me," then you are correct. If you believe that "This is an opportunity to be outside of my comfort zone," then you are also correct.

Neither one is more or less true, but each thought will affect you in very different ways. Which one should you choose to follow?

The answer is obvious.

No one would consciously choose to feel worse in this situation, but it does happen sometimes. The reason is that many of us forfeit our ability to choose the response by automatically choosing the dark side—the default. However, as we become more aware, we have a greater ability to choose healthy, empowering thoughts.

Do you think making this positive choice is worth a little of your time and attention?

KEY POINTS

1. You are not your thoughts. You are the space in which they arise.
2. Emotions are the driving force behind communication.
3. Writing down negative thoughts is like creating antivirus software.
4. "A belief is nothing more than a thought we keep thinking" (Hicks).
5. Increased awareness = increased ability to choose empowering beliefs.
6. "Everything is true, but some truths are more limited than others" (Ramtha, *The White Book*).
7. The truth is 100% dependent on the meaning we attach to it.

Clearing Out Space: Exercises

The exercises in this section are designed to help you align your communication with your deepest intentions. Clearing out space gets easier over time, but it is a never-ending process. The more aware we become, the slicker the ego gets at slipping in the back door. So we must continue to upgrade our anti-virus software. No matter how far we have come, there are always more layers to shed and new levels of joy to experience.

Experiencing the lower energy level of the ego brings on familiar feelings. In my experience, it is usually a sense of "blah," struggle, or frustration. The more aware you become of how your particular ego feels and operates, the less likely you will be to fall into its traps.

These exercises come from slightly different angles but are designed to help you upgrade your software for clinical success. I recommend keeping them on file and repeating them as you progress in your journey.

EXERCISE #1: I AM NOT THE "VOICE" THAT SAYS . . .

I once heard Eckhart Tolle say, "The best way to know who you are is to know who you are not."

Attempting to know who we are through the thinking brain is a wild goose chase. The voice in the head will try to convince us otherwise, but the mental ideas and images we have about ourselves have nothing to do with our real identity.

The voice in the head is *not* who we are, but it does determine who we are **being** in this world. Once we break our identification with it, we become free to **choose** thoughts and beliefs that will create more fruitful and enjoyable life experiences.

I had a profound aha! moment a few years ago when I thought, I could continue to be the same struggling guy I am or I could be a happy-go-lucky guy. But neither one is the real me. They are just alternate personas that I could choose to be.

I am now generally happier because I am more empowered (aware) to choose wisely. My internal dialogue is much more positive, but it is still not the real me. I have simply learned to use it to my advantage, instead of being its #1 victim.

I recommend keeping a running **"I am Not the 'Voice' that Says . . ."** list. Add as many self-limiting thoughts as you can identify. Remember, just like computer viruses, the negative thoughts are very good at hiding, so writing them down as they arise can be very helpful.

This is a simple but very powerful technique for making room for empowering thoughts. Here is an example of how to get started.

I Am Not the "Voice" that Says . . .

1. I am not good enough.
2. I have to be perfect.
3. I am not smart enough.
4. I can't do it.
5. I am supposed to know everything.

The more specific you can be, the better. Remember, when you say, "I'm NOT the voice," you are NOT lying—the voice is just an old program. All you are doing is making room to upgrade your system.

EXERCISE #2: OLD SELF TO IDEAL SELF

Dr. Joe recommended this exercise after I asked him the following question: "Do we reach a point where we have to stop labeling everything (e.g., "There is my anxiety.")? It seems that labeling can lead to analysis that causes even more problems. Is this true?"

Dr. Joe agreed that we eventually do need to stop labeling everything. But he also said that we must first become aware of the many subtle ways we get sucked in without our awareness. The ego tends to become cleverer as we evolve, and it will do anything to keep the internal conversation alive. **Analyzing and trying to figure things out mentally is one of its most seductive traps**.

One of Dr. Joe's basic messages is that *we go from thinking to doing to being*. Research shows that 90% of our thoughts are unconscious. We are often unaware of the thoughts that reinforce identification with certain emotions and behaviors.

Here is an example. Many people believe that "life is stressful." They wake up every day with a general mindset of "I just want to get through the day."

The morning traffic automatically triggers frustration and reactivity, which they take out on other drivers. When they get to work, they react negatively to their "toxic boss," then they overact when their lunch order is wrong. Through daily repetition of this pattern, many people become "**stress**." It is **not** who these people really are, but it is who they are **being** on a regular basis.

The next exercise is a great way to break this cycle and to empower yourself to become whomever you want to be. Feel free to structure the exercise however you like. Start with listing character traits and specific thoughts and behaviors that reinforce that trait, going from negative to positive.

This exercise is about becoming more familiar with the qualities you do and do not want to emulate. I recommend listing several thoughts and behaviors for each trait (I included a couple to get you started).

Example:

Old-Self Trait: Anxiety

Thoughts: "What if I make a mistake?"

Behaviors: I get tense, rigid, and hesitant in planning and execution.

New-Self Trait: Self-assured

Thoughts: "I think I can do it, and if I need help, I will ask. I do not have to be perfect."

Behaviors: I do my best and ask for help as needed.

This exercise is very useful because it illustrates the connections between the thoughts, behaviors, and personality traits that we embody. I recommend giving this exercise a lot of attention.

EXERCISE 3: "SCREENWRITING"—OLD SELF, NEW SELF

This exercise is similar to exercise #2 but is easier to implement on the fly, as we become more familiar with our patterns.

Pretend you are the screenwriter of your own story (which you really are, by the way), and start asking the questions, "What is my old self saying right now? What would my new self say?"

Notice I did not say, "What am *I* saying right now?"

Whether it is positive or negative, **you** are **not** the self (voice in your head). Approaching the situation from the outside in this way makes it less personal and easier to implement.

If I practiced this during my clinical rotations, it would have sounded like:

"My old self is saying I have to be perfect, but my new self would say just relax and do the best I can."

"My old self is saying I am supposed to know everything already, but my new self would say I am new and learning. I am not supposed to know everything."

"My old self is saying my client knows I am clueless, but my new self would say they care most about me doing my best and giving them my full attention."

EXERCISE #4: UPGRADING BELIEFS

The book *The Law of Attraction* explains that a belief is nothing more than a thought we keep thinking. Behind every negative thought is a belief that is driving and reinforcing negative patterns of thinking.

Think of beliefs like the foundation of a house. When we take out the foundation, the entire house falls. Becoming familiar with specific negative thoughts is valuable (like clearing out the rubble). It is also helpful to expose limiting beliefs that support them.

This exercise addresses both becoming familiar with and exposing the negatives while providing a technique for reprogramming new beliefs into the brain and body.

Here are a few examples to help you get started.

What Negative Thought am I thinking? "I'll never be able to do it."

What do I believe when I think this thought? "I'm not good enough."

What Conscious Thought do I want to choose instead? "I'm going to give it my best shot."

What do I want to program myself to believe? "I am good enough."

Upgrading Your Software: Recommended/Related Resources

1. *The Biology of Belief* (Lipton)
2. *Breaking the Habit of Being Yourself* (Dispenza)
3. *The Law of Attraction* (Hicks)

LOOKING IN THE MIRROR

Pam Trained Her "Inner Puppy" & Her Dog

My colleague Pam is a young, smart, talented, delightful person. After being exposed to the power of these teachings, she said, "Oh my God! Every OT in the world needs to learn this!"

It wasn't too long before she started openly admitting that she was not practicing what she was preaching. She shared with me, "I was teaching the importance of thinking positive and not overreacting, and I wasn't practicing that in my own life."

She became progressively more introspective and started noticing how her thoughts affected her mood and her behavior. One day, she told her group a great story about her dog Hendrix.

Pam related: "I started noticing how nervous I was when passing people during walks with Hendrix. He's the sweetest dog, but many people are scared of pitbulls. I had this recurring thought, 'What if Hendrix scares someone?' But then I started questioning this nonsense and **choosing** thoughts like, 'He's a really calm dog. He's never threatened anyone. Plenty of people love his breed.' Hendrix started doing *so much better* when I improved my energy by changing my thought process."

I have a lot of respect for Pam, because in addition to training her "Inner Puppy," she had also begun building her dog-training knowledge before she rescued Hendrix. She read books, consulted dog trainers, and focused on a particular goal (owning a well-trained dog). It is no surprise that she owns a well-trained dog that everyone loves.

She did this by downloading/programming her "Dog Training Software," but her success would not have been possible without her being equally committed to training her "Inner Puppy" by choosing more empowering thoughts.

CHAPTER 6

REBOOTING YOUR SYSTEM

Do you find yourself complaining despite *knowing* that it is only making your life more difficult? Don't feel bad; we are all guilty of this at times.

Understanding the Power of Acceptance

Everyone knows "It is what it is," but we often resist "what is" when we don't like it. The reason is that complaining temporarily eases pain (numbs emotion) while removing any sense of personal responsibility.

Resisting also reaffirms our ego's sense of identity by reinforcing our identification with our emotions, beliefs, and opinions (e.g., "I am right!" or "This shouldn't be this way!").

Remember, this is *not* a conscious process. No one stops and says, "I am going to resist this because it feels good."

This habit is more common than you might think. Many of us spend a great deal of our waking life unconscious, resisting the reality of the present moment. I remember hearing this for the first time and thinking, Yes, that's right; people (not me) are unconscious so much of the time.

I did not realize how quickly I projected my unconsciousness onto others—it was a convenient distraction. Looking internally requires a sense of courage and humility, but it is well worth the exploration.

Acceptance: A Non-Doing Process

Acceptance is a difficult concept to explain because it requires no effort. Instead of "doing" (trying to get rid of) something, acceptance requires us to "not do." It requires us to let go, trust, and be the space that can absorb the clouds.

It feels great to just "**be** there" for someone, doesn't it? Not saying anything, judging them, or giving them advice, just being a calm presence that supports them in fully being with their feelings.

Many of us can be that safe space for others but not so much for ourselves. The good news is that the formula is the same, and it has everything to do with acceptance.

Defining Acceptance

Acceptance is *not* a passive process where we say to ourselves, "This is just the way it is, and there is nothing I can do to change the situation."

Acceptance *is* an active, yet "non-doing" process of compassionately (i.e., without judgment) attending to the present moment and simply "being the space" for the emotional clouds we are experiencing.

Acceptance allows the clouds to clear, enabling us to access our own wisdom and greatest intelligence. We can then naturally be guided toward actions that will improve the situation we are experiencing.

Radical Acceptance

Radical Acceptance by Tara Brach is a great resource for learning how to break patterns of resistance. She explains that Radical Acceptance has two inseparable qualities of attention: mindfulness and compassion. "Like two wings of a bird, we need them both in their fullest expression to fly and be free."

If we are not mindful, we remain ignorant. But if we are too mindful, we become too analytical. If we are not compassionate, we blame others (or beat up ourselves). But if we are too compassionate, then we are prone to take on the victim mode, which can be equally destructive. The focus is to find the perfect blending of the two.

The following illustrates the two forms of acceptance:

1. Non-Radical Acceptance: "I'm such an idiot! I can't believe I just did that again. I just can't do this anymore!"

Clearly there is no compassion, no consciousness here; we are just beating ourselves up, which is unlikely to result in an improved mood or performance.

2. Radical Acceptance: "Oh man . . . (breathing, "space," etc.) I can't believe I just did that. I feel horrible about it, and now I have to pay the consequences. But I didn't mean to, so I'm going to learn from this so that I don't make the same mistake again."

We are not sugarcoating anything. We are not trying to pretend we feel good when we don't; we simply don't beat ourselves up for being human.

Acceptance Is a Process of Letting Go

Habitual resistance results in the buildup of a great deal of internal pressure. Just like shaking and then opening that soda bottle, we have to slowly untwist the cap and allow the pressure to escape gradually. Practicing acceptance is like patiently holding the bottle, allowing the built-up pressure to settle. Only then can we begin the process of slowly untwisting the cap.

The first step to resolving any issue is admitting that one exists. Habitual resistance is so common that it can be difficult to notice (feel), even when we are committed to practicing acceptance.

"How do I know if I've truly accepted something?" is a great question. The answer is: "If I have truly accepted something, it is a nonissue. It brings up no emotional charge."

It is much easier to accept that we have not fully accepted something than it is to ignore resistance—this takes a lot of energy. Acceptance requires courage and humility, but the reward—freedom from suffering—is invaluable.

Carl Jung understood this when he said: "We cannot change anything until we accept it. Condemnation does not liberate; it oppresses."

The following Key Points and exercises can help you get started on your acceptance journey.

KEY POINTS

1. Acceptance results in an unmistakable sign of inner peace. (Tolle, *Power of Now*)

2. Acceptance is an active process of "non-doing."

3. Acceptance = "Being the Space" (i.e., just being there) for ourselves.

4. Acceptance requires a sense of honesty, humility, and courage.

5. Acceptance often happens over time.

6. The more we accept, the more peace we experience. (Brach)

7. Acceptance is a compassionate, not forceful, process.

8. Acceptance is a skill we can learn.

Getting Honest with Ourselves: What Am I Resisting?

Acceptance is an ongoing process that requires honesty about past and current issues. Creating lists of things you intuitively know that need your compassionate attention (acceptance) is a good way to start. Below are examples of how you can begin.

What are my past issues that require acceptance?

1. I worry about performance because _____.

2. I am still holding resentment toward _____.

3. I do not believe I am worthy of _____.

4. I still have not gotten over my relationship with _____.

5. I am paralyzed by fear, which keeps me from _____.

6. I do not like myself because of _____.

7. I carry a lot of anger about _____.

8. I cover up _____ by _____.

9. I seek approval because _____.

10. I don't express my needs and feelings because _____.

11. _____ has been keeping me from experiencing more joy my whole life.

What are ongoing issues that require acceptance?

1. I blame _____ for being in a bad mood.

2. I am addicted to _____.

3. I judge people for _____ because it makes me feel better about myself.

4. I care too much about what other people think about _____.

5. I know I should start _____.

6. I get really passive-aggressive about _____.

7. I put other people's needs before my own at the expense of my own well-being.

8. I focus more on trying to change other people than on working on myself.

9. I sabotage myself by _____.

10. I rely on _____ way too much.

Again, these are just examples. We must each create our own lists and keep adding to them as we move forward. This is a great way to release pressure and may lead to actions that prevent the build up in the first place.

The following is a list of Acceptance/Releasing Pressure actions, along with a brief explanation of why they are effective.

Acceptance/Releasing Pressure Actions

1. <u>Cathartic Letter Writing</u>: This is a process of writing emotional letters (angry, sad, resentful, etc.) with the intention of releasing negative energy in a healthy way. We do not send the letters to anyone. In fact, burning them can be an effective ritual that can be helpful in releasing, letting go, and then finding acceptance. We want to get "raw" when writing these letters, for the sole

intention of releasing pent-up negative energy and facilitating the process of acceptance.

2. "The Elephant in the Room" Conversations: Avoiding conflict and uncomfortable conversation is at the root of most suffering. Stepping up to the plate and initiating real conversations is one of the healthiest actions we can take. This can be difficult to do, but it is nothing compared to the energy it takes to pretend everything is fine when it is not. "The Elephant in the Room" conversations are not about achieving a particular result. These conversations are about acting with integrity and speaking our truth. It is an action of high integrity that often leads to positive change and a stronger sense of self.

Rebooting Your System: Recommended Related Resources

1. *Broken Open* (Lesser)
2. *Daring Greatly* (Brown)
3. *Radical Acceptance* (Brach)
4. *The Dark Side of Light Chasers* (Ford)
5. *The Power of Now* (Tolle)
6. Tara Brach's Free Podcast (I recommend browsing for specific topics/titles that interest you.)

LOOKING IN THE MIRROR

The Power of Accepting "What Is"

Lisa beat all the odds. As a teenage parent and single mom, she raised three children, managed to work full time, and was very close to earning her bachelor's degree. She was a kind, strong, and determined woman who wanted the very best for her children.

A diagnosis of multiple sclerosis in her early forties forced her to slow down for the first time in her life. As you can imagine, it was very difficult for her to accept that her life had changed. She did what many of us would do in her situation: she resisted the truth.

I didn't realize how much emotional pain she was in until we had a one-on-one session. She was very good at pretending that everything was okay, even though she was hurting inside. I learned that she woke up crying every morning. I felt so bad for her and desperately wanted to help; yet I intuitively knew there was nothing I could do. She needed to accept "what is," and I could not do that for her. All I could "do" was be (the space) there for her. We sat in silence together for a few minutes. It was initially uncomfortable for me (I was used to doing something to help), but then it just began to feel right. No words can adequately describe the experience, but it was one of the deepest connections I have ever shared with another person.

The next day, Lisa looked much better. Her mood had improved (from 2/10 to 6/10), and she had told herself, "No, not today," that morning when feeling the urge to cry. She recognized that her daily crying sessions were no longer productive—they were keeping her stuck. Her physical symptoms (gait and speech) started improving, and her mood progressively brightened. She looked like a new person by the time she was discharged. On her last day, I asked her, "What turned things around for you?" She replied, "It was that session we had; that was the moment I accepted my illness."

CHAPTER 7

CLEARING COOKIES: USING ENERGY TO STAY "IN THE ZONE"

I mentioned earlier that we are made of 99.999% empty space, or energy. I struggled for so many years because I did not understand or recognize this fact. I remained "zoomed in" on my much smaller physical self, ignoring the greater part of my identity. I progressed in some respects, but I never felt at home with myself and usually felt a sense of unease.

I was also consumed by the roles I played (coach, the personal-growth guy, etc.), and was convinced that I was personally responsible ("I did that!") for my successes.

This was especially the case when it came to my own personal transformation. So, I was both defensive and disturbed the first time I heard Eckhart Tolle say, "We can't transform ourselves. All we can do is create the space so that it can happen." I thought, What do you mean? I've been transforming myself for years!

Now I understand. I never transformed myself; I just created space so that the transformation could happen. I accomplished this by exploring the variety of techniques included in this book that helped me become more present. I did not realize at the time that I was practicing the ultimate form of Energy Medicine—presence.

We are fortunate to have a variety of Energy Medicine modalities, including acupuncture, Qigong, yoga, Zero Balancing, and Reiki, all of which have value. But their effects are limited without a commitment of making presence our highest priority.

Here is why.

Any one of the modalities mentioned above will likely elicit a more emotionally balanced state. However, in many cases, the peaceful feeling quickly becomes a distant memory. The reason is that we often return to the same thought process that created the energy blocks (which were removed by the treatment) in the first place. And when this happens, we often are not aware enough to *know*—"Wait, I'm getting out of balance, it's time for another yoga class."

I was guilty of this for several years, which is why I kept struggling. I was always busy looking for the next "thing" to make me feel better. In the meantime, I was missing the most important piece of the puzzle— being present.

The single most powerful form of Energy Medicine is learning how to pay attention to the present moment. The positive feelings we get from yoga, Qigong, acupuncture, etc. are *not dependent* on any of those modalities; they just make becoming present easier. The only thing that can make us "stay" is our attention.

Energy Medicine modalities are very valuable. They can facilitate and support us in maintaining a healthy and balanced life. We just need to understand that they are tools—not magic bullets.

Paying attention to how we are paying attention is the closest thing to a magic bullet. Attention to the present moment naturally keeps us in tune with our energy. It is what enables us to be **aware** of when and how we can benefit from a particular Energy Medicine modality.

People often mistake what I do with teaching a path, but this is not the case. I teach a knowledge base that enables people to trust their intuition and choose their own path. There are many ways to become more rooted in the present moment; we each must find our own way.

Managing our energy on a moment-by-moment basis (paying attention) *is* what makes this possible.

I spent seven years ignoring the impact of attention and energy until I was introduced to Karl Ardo, a Qigong master and Zero Balancing practitioner. He was the first person to explain that this is more than an intellectual process.

He said: "You're just stuck in your left brain, and you need to find balance. Qigong and Zero Balancing are tools that can help, but ultimately, it's really about letting go and trusting."

A Little Exercise that Opened My Eyes

Karl immediately had my attention when he showed me a basic Qigong technique. I encourage you to try it on your own. He said: "Raise your arms out to the side as you normally would. Now, raise them pretending there are strings on your wrists that a puppeteer is pulling. Inhale as you go up and exhale as you go down. Did you notice a difference?"

The difference was obvious to me. He explained that the initial motions were just mechanical, muscular movements, with no life or energy. The subsequent **conscious** movements were not just psychologically lighter; they actually were lighter. The motions took less effort and felt more fluid with the puppeteer image in mind. Karl explained that I was creating energy with this latter type of motion.

Many of us are so busy with life and live so unconsciously and mechanically that we forget about the energy that makes everything possible. Energy Medicine modalities can be helpful because they remove energy blocks—they "un-kink the hose" and allow the energy to flow freely.

KEY POINTS

1. The greater part of who we are is energy.
2. Paying attention is the foundation of Energy Medicine.
3. Energy Medicine can remove emotional/energy blocks.
4. Energy Medicine keeps our energy flowing more efficiently.
5. The cells of the body are 100 times more receptive to energy than to chemicals (Dispenza, *You Are the Placebo*). This is why Energy Medicine should not be considered alternative.

Meditation—It's NOT Just about Sitting with Your Eyes Closed

Meditation is a process of observing without judgment, with your eyes closed or open.

Formal Meditation

Many people think meditation is just about sitting with your eyes closed while focusing on your breathing. That is what you might call Formal Meditation, which is just one of many meditation options. The general purpose of Formal Meditation is simply to observe or watch your thoughts (like a ticker on a TV screen) without reacting to them.

As you know, many of us become consumed by our thoughts and get sucked into analyzing them, thereby creating confusion and stress. Formal Meditation is the practice of training ourselves to notice without judgment ("Oh, I'm thinking again"), and then gently guiding ourselves back ("Let me refocus on my breath") to the present moment. Formal Meditation exercises our focus muscle—the frontal lobe.

Regular practice (for example, a half hour every day) can be helpful, like a training camp for your life. If you catch yourself drifting and return to the present moment multiple times during your meditation, you will be more likely to stay focused throughout the day—a key component of your clinical success.

Meditation will make your brain healthier, regardless of which type of meditation you choose to practice. Below is a list of several additional meditation exercises you can explore.

Tara Brach is a therapist and an excellent meditation instructor. Her website offers a great deal of free education as well as countless guided meditations that can support your practice.

Meditation through Activity

If you do not feel ready to sit with your eyes closed, you can also practice meditation through activity. All you have to do is pay closer attention to your senses as you complete activities throughout your day.

It is best to start with one activity, like brushing your teeth or taking a shower. Simply observe the sensations you feel as you complete the mundane task. You will quickly notice that the task is far from mundane when you are actually paying attention. Here is an example of something you can try in the shower.

Notice the temperature of the water, the beads of water dripping, the smooth feeling of the soap, the smell of the shampoo, the sounds of water, your breathing as you take it all in, etc.

There is no right or wrong way to meditate through activity. It is simply to consciously complete the activity rather than just do it mechanically. The difference in the experience is invaluable, especially when it is an activity you typically may not enjoy. For example, washing dishes is not my favorite job, but I actually *enjoy* doing it when I am paying attention.

"Feeling I" (Worth Discussing Again!)

The greater part of who we are is energy. Paying attention to the energy field in the body is a way to stay connected to the real you (Tolle). It is also a way to reduce the stress-producing internal dialogue.

Here is how to do it. Close your eyes and feel the energy in your hands. It might be helpful to ask yourself, "How can I know my hands are there without looking at them?" You will notice you can feel them. Once you can sense the energy, repeat the following statement (internally or aloud) for three minutes: "I am this feeling . . . this feeling is me . . . I am this feeling . . . this feeling is me."

"Feeling I" will bring you into a state of peace. It will also establish a new connection in your brain—"I am Energy." In other words, you will break your identification with the mental story of your life that causes unnecessary stress.

Acupuncture

Acupuncture practitioners place small needles where energy blocks exist, to facilitate the process of moving energy. The very short duration of a pinch you may feel when the needles are inserted is well worth the long-term benefits of acupuncture. Acupuncturists also tend to be calm, resourceful, and connected people who offer valuable, practical wisdom as well.

Emotional Freedom Technique (EFT)

Emotional Freedom Technique (EFT) is a simple but powerful form of Energy Medicine that you can learn to do independently. Many forms of EFT exist, but they all involve tapping on acupressure points to free up energy and process emotion.

Imagine having a brand new TV with a severed HDMI cord. It is not going to work because the signal cannot be transmitted properly. The same is true when we are stuck emotionally.

EFT is a skill you can learn to do independently, but investing in a few sessions with a certified EFT practitioner can save you a lot of time and energy.

A wealth of free information and lists of EFT providers can be found on the Internet, including http://www.thetappingsolution.com, http://www.carollook.com, and http://www.eftuniverse.com. You can also find countless free videos on YouTube.

Qigong

Qigong (pronounced *chee-gong*) is a movement meditation. Karl Ardo, who introduced me to it, named his practice "Moving in Stillness," because it is a process of learning to "still" the mind while moving the body. A variety of forms of Qigong exist. I recommend starting with an introductory medical Qigong class, which will give you a solid foundation for continuing Qigong meditation. Research has shown many profound physical and mental benefits of Qigong. It literally means "Life Energy Cultivation."

Qigong for Runners

If you like running, you will likely find chirunning very helpful. It is a specific technique for bringing consciousness (energy) into your runs, making them easier and more natural (less exerting).

Here is Karl's explanation.

"Imagine having a stream of energy flowing from between your shoulder blades out to the center of your chest. As you run, lean forward about a half inch (as if you're about to fall), and imagine the energy creating a circular motion, like pedaling a bicycle. The consciousness of that image will create a flow of energy that will propel you with much greater ease."

Consider the difference between average marathon runners and Kenyan runners. Average runners run mechanically, whereas Kenyan runners appear to float on air. In a way, that is what they are doing, and chirunning is a skill any runner can learn.

Miscellaneous Energy Medicine Forms

The following is a list of additional modalities worth exploring. This is in no way a complete list. I recommend doing your own research and finding those forms that resonate with you. You are likely to find other options as you create your own recipe for Energy Medicine practices.

1. Yoga
2. Reiki
3. Rolfing
4. Guided Imagery
5. Aromatherapy
6. Sound Healing (www.tomkenyon.com)
7. Progressive Muscle Relaxation
8. Crystal Healing
9. Chanting Therapy

LOOKING IN THE MIRROR

It's All about Balance

Several years ago, I went through a very rough time. Intellectually, I knew everything I should do, but I was stuck emotionally. I could present myself as the expert, but I could not walk the talk. I was an expert at suppressing my emotions by using my left analytical brain.

This habit became progressively more difficult to hide as things started rising to the surface. I could no longer intellectualize myself into a "good" mood. I consulted a colleague who told me, "You know the inner workings of the clock so well that it screws you up."

She was right; it was time to find balance in my life. I started giving equal (if not more) attention to energy modalities, such as Qigong, meditation, yoga, Reiki, and others. I did not realize it at the time but this is when I really started practicing "Presence."

Professionally, a funny thing started happening. I began providing better care with less effort. It wasn't natural at first. In fact, I felt very uncomfortable slowing down and choosing my words more carefully. Nevertheless, I persisted, and before long I began receiving comments like, "You're so calm, which helps me relax."

I wasn't necessarily saying or teaching anything different, yet clients seemed to receive and implement what I was sharing on a more consistent basis. I next realized that **the words we choose mean little; it's the energy in which they are delivered that matters the most.**

I share this story because I believe (as discussed) that there is a large imbalance between "being" and "doing" in our healthcare system. This creates a great deal of stress, which negatively impacts the quality of care we deliver.

Energy Medicine modalities can help you facilitate and maintain the highest quality of energy—a key component to optimizing your performance.

CHAPTER 8

KEEPING YOUR SYSTEM UPDATED

Change is the process of breaking old habits and creating new ones. It occurs over time with a great deal of practice. Remember, as Dr. Joe teaches, we must practice until "the body knows better than the mind"—until being present becomes our new habit.

With a concentrated effort, developing this new habit can happen faster than you might think. Understanding the process of change and becoming familiar with the common stumbling blocks can make it easier to create new habits.

Dr. Joe describes the four types of competence in his book *Evolve Your Brain: The Science of Changing Your Mind,* which relates to our discussion. Let's see how a "road rager" becomes a "Zen driver" using Dr. Joe's teaching combined with what we have learned.

Creating New Habits: The Four Types of Competence

1. Unconsciously Incompetent: At this stage, we are not aware that a problem exists. This is the "**I am a road rager** and I can't change." We may be aware of the problem on some level, but we are so **identified** with it that we cannot envision the possibility of change.

2. Consciously Incompetent: At this stage, we are now aware of the problem but don't have the skill(s) for changing the behavior. This is the "I really have to learn how to remain calm in traffic" stage.

3. <u>Consciously Competent</u>: At this stage, we are actively learning. We can remain calm in traffic but it takes a fair amount of conscious intention and energy to do so. We can easily lose it if we are not paying attention. The length of time we remain in this phase depends on factors like

- the level of emotional attachment to the behavior;
- how long we've been doing it;
- the level of commitment to change; and
- most important, our ability to create the space so the outdated habit can dissolve on its own. This is a delicate process of learning to let go and to trust, instead of holding onto the thought processes that are like training wheels on a bicycle. For example, the "road rager" might start off by reminding himself to just relax, but eventually he must become relaxed. As Dr. Joe teaches, we go from thinking to doing to being.

4. <u>Unconsciously Competent</u>: At this stage, we have now acquired a new habit. The body knows better than the mind. We no longer have to think about this particular skill, it just happens naturally. The "road rager" has now become a "Zen driver."

Change Is NOT Supposed to Be Easy

Change is not supposed to be easy, but in the long run, it is easier than desperately trying to stay in the comfort zone. As the saying goes, the butterfly is not meant to stay in its cocoon.

Deepak Chopra describes the "Law of Least Effort" in his book *The*

Seven Spiritual Laws of Success. As the name implies, ideally, we should take whatever action requires the least amount of effort.

I ask clients this unusual hypothetical question: "Would you rather have me slap you in the face really hard one time or gently pat you on your face for an hour?"

Everyone always says, "Just get it over with quickly."

Change operates in a similar way. In the short run, it stings, but it's hardly anything compared to the chronic long-term pain we create for ourselves by resisting change.

Transitioning from being "consciously competent" to "unconsciously competent" can be an arduous process, requiring a great deal of time and energy. Accepting that this is a normal part of the process can make it considerably easier.

Remember, this is not supposed to be easy, and it is not about having to be perfect. It is about becoming the master of your mind and body. It requires discipline and a plan of action.

Here are some guidelines for creating a self-care program that will work for you.

KEY POINTS

1. Change is not supposed to be easy. Begin with an appreciation of this.
2. Establishing rituals/habits is an essential component of change.
3. Create your own recipe for practices that work for you.
4. "It is about progress, not perfection." (Tony Robbins)
5. Paying attention = the foundation for positive change.

6. The process of evolving/changing never stops.

7. Suffering is the result of resisting your natural evolution.

8. "Staying" present gets easier over time.

The Three Essentials: Ingredients

The Three Essentials are fundamental to a successful plan. Regardless of the specific activities you choose to incorporate, the following will help you maintain a sense of balance that will lead to inner peace and optimal performance.

1. Establishing Rituals/Habits: Staying present can be challenging, even if doing so is a priority. But, if staying present is not your priority, remaining so is virtually impossible. Even though we must decide what works for us, it is important to recognize that creating rituals is essential to staying present. Imagine the difference between getting up and racing to work versus giving yourself a half hour to get calm and centered before you start your day. The energy we create in the morning can set the tone for the entire day. Evening rituals that include winding down, reflecting, and learning from the day's experiences can also be effective. Again, you must decide what works best for you.

   Personally, I do not like a lot of structure, so I frequently vary my rituals. But I take healthy actions every morning to prep myself for the day. This may include inspirational videos/music, meditation, use of affirmations, spending quality time with my pets, and other actions. I also settle down at night and set my intention of how I want to sleep and wake up the next day.

I was not always committed to such a structure, and I struggled more than was necessary. Do yourself a favor, and start creating and committing to your own rituals as soon as possible.

2. <u>Remember the Three Most Important Things</u>: SEE CHAPTER 3

3. <u>Conscious Movement</u>: We miss out on the beauty that surrounds us each and every moment when we are not paying attention. Being open to our senses is one of the easiest and most powerful tools for staying in the present moment. It naturally facilitates Open-Focus Attention—a key to staying in the zone.

Creating Your Self-Care Program

Here are the 10 most important strategies to consider when developing your program. I use all of them regularly but generally not on the same day. My body (when I am paying attention) usually tells me what strategy is needed in any given moment. Trust your gut—it is much smarter than your thinking brain.

1. <u>Exercise/Posture/Breathing</u>: Most of us are familiar with the health benefits of each of these, yet many of us neglect our bodies. We underestimate the impact that poor breathing and bad posture have on the flow of energy. Proper breathing, ergonomically correct posture, and exercise are essential to optimal physical and mental health. Amy Cuddy's TED Talk on body language is **powerful** and worth watching.

2. <u>Exploring New Knowledge</u>: Life-changing information that can be used to facilitate optimal physical and mental health is released daily, and it has never been cheaper or easier to access.

Imagine how different your life would be in a year if you devoted an hour each day to exploring personal growth materials instead of indulging in too much trash (reality TV, social media, etc.). I am not suggesting that we give up our guilty pleasures but just that we need to understand the importance of striking a better balance. One of my favorite practices is exercising while listening to inspirational materials.

3. <u>Social Supports/Accountability</u>: The path of personal growth can be lonely at times. Many people are not yet on the path and still choose short-term gratification over long-term fulfillment. You may find that some of the people you are close to may not understand or be interested in your journey. They may even (unconsciously) attempt to restrain you to make themselves feel more comfortable.

   For example, my friend's brother said to her, "You're not being a good sister," when she refused to listen to his complaints about their parents. He secretly felt bad about his behavior, but it was easier (in the short term) to blame her rather than to look internally. Remember, this is not a conscious process.

   I have a great family and many friends, but I have only a select few with whom I share my journey of personal growth. These people are compassionate, non-judgmental, direct, honest, and real. They hold me accountable to a high standard of behavior, and I do the same for them.

   Finding at least one person that you can be completely real with is invaluable.

4. <u>Energy Medicine</u>: (SEE CHAPTER 7) Energy Medicine modalities can facilitate the process of change. Do your own research, and trust the modalities (if any) that feel right to you. You may get lucky and meet someone who can be of great support (as I was when I met Karl).

5. <u>Formal Meditation</u>: Everything discussed in this book is about meditation—which is synonymous with being aware. You do not have to sit down with your eyes closed to reap the benefits. But if you want to be "in the zone" more often, I highly recommend starting a formal meditation practice. This is becoming increasingly popular for good reason—it works! You can choose from a countless list of teachers, approaches, and resources. If you are not sure where to start, Tara Brach is a safe bet.

6. <u>Learning Journaling</u>: This is a process of self-reflection where you take an objective (judgment-free) look at your performance. This is not about grading yourself. It is about celebrating your successes and learning from your mistakes. Answering the following questions is a good way to structure your Learning Journal.

   "What did I do well today? How did I stay on track? What helped me to stay conscious? What new results/experiences did I create? Where did I fall off track? How can I do better next time? What did I learn today?"

   Noticing and documenting even the smallest changes in behavior is very important. The reason is that many of us are conditioned to look at what we did wrong instead of what we did right ("I would have gotten 100% on the exam if I didn't miss that easy question!").

Celebrating our successes wires us neurologically to replicate the behavior. This is the reason babies and dogs respond so well to praise. It is not about stroking the ego; it is about acknowledging our efforts, no matter how small or big.

7. Affirmations: These are positive statements of intent that work like advertisements. We eventually buy (believe) whatever thoughts we keep repeating. Examples include "I am confident" and "I can do it."

    Many people find affirmations ineffective, and here's why. They believe that they **have to say them** for them to be true. Remember, everything is true—what we believe is just a matter of conditioning.

    The thought "I will be (fill in quality) one day if I keep saying this" is a huge trap. It's the ego in disguise attempting to sabotage our efforts.

    Affirmations become powerful when they are infused with who we are, namely "energy." We can begin to encode new beliefs with much greater ease. I have included a supplement with Affirmation Guidelines at the end of this chapter to help you get started.

8. Segment Intention Setting (Hicks): Take "mini time-outs" to set clear intentions for any given activity, a powerful way to create positive karma. As Hicks teaches, "You are pre-paving your future."

Here are some examples.

- Driving: "My intention is to drive safely and peacefully to my destination."

- Phone: "My intention is to have a peaceful, authentic conversation."

- Important Project: "My intention is to be joyfully focused as I give this project my best effort."

- Sleeping: "My intention is to have a restful night and wake up feeling energized and inspired."

- Competition: "My intention is to remain joyfully focused as I do my best to win."

Imagine the difference this could have on the outcomes of all of these activities.

9. Old Self Versus New Self: (SEE CHAPTER 5)

10. Gratitude Journaling and Active Appreciation: I once heard Dr. Joe say, "When you ask a person who is in a state of gratitude why they can't have something they want, they won't be able to give you an answer. The subconscious mind, which holds onto the negative tapes, literally shuts down."

Gratitude Journaling is very powerful. We often do not fully appreciate everything we take for granted. Last year, I allowed the thought "I don't feel like working out" to prevent me from exercising. It wasn't until I sustained an injury and temporarily (thankfully) lost the ability to exercise that I appreciated the gift of being able to do so.

The value of focusing on reasons we have to be grateful

is immeasurable. It is also a way to remain present. However, practicing Active Appreciation is even more important.

Active Appreciation is a process of asking, **"What can I appreciate/feel grateful for right now?"** whenever we find ourselves in a negative state.

Affirmation Guidelines

Affirmation Facts

1. They work. It is normal not to believe this at first, but it will help to work your way up to more positive programs. For example, if your current program is "I hate myself," saying "I love myself" will be too much of a leap. "I have some positive qualities" might be a more reasonable place to start.

2. They require repetition.

3. They feel great when repeated from your core.

4. How Do I Choose My Affirmations? Pick statements that address specific areas of need. Here are a few examples.

    A. Perfectionism: "I allow myself to be imperfect."

    B. Complaining: "I take responsibility for how I feel."

    C. Approval Seeking: "I don't care what other people think."

A good rule of thumb is if it *feels* right to you, then it is right. Be open and flexible to changing your "affirmation play list." Just like music, different "songs" apply, depending on your mood in any given moment.

Summary

Now it is up to you. Until you put this information into practice, it's all just nice theory. You must implement what you have learned to experience the true value of these important lessons. Ironically, the more wisdom you gain, the less you will need the information contained in this book, or anywhere else for that matter. Everything you need to know is already within you—all you have to do is get out of the way.

From Depression to Empowerment

Rita came into our program as a very timid, depressed woman. Initially, she was Unconsciously Incompetent—she really could not see that change was possible. It didn't take her long to become Consciously Incompetent, meaning she understood that she could change but had no idea how to get started. Even though she regularly attended the program, she wasn't very engaged and didn't appear motivated, hardly saying a word to anyone. Intellectually, she *knew* what she needed to do, but she couldn't get started. I was beginning to doubt her level of commitment when one day she surprised me.

I always ask clients to share examples in their life of when they felt themselves becoming more aware and making empowered choices, no matter how small. Rita (reluctantly) shared, "I did something different this weekend. Normally, I isolate myself during family functions. I wanted to, but I forced myself to stay outside with everyone. I didn't say much, but at least I didn't isolate myself." This was a *huge* shift for her that I don't believe she fully appreciated until we talked about the process of change. The tendency, especially for those who are hard on themselves, is to downplay progress. ("It's no big deal.") It's their subtle way of reinforcing their "old self."

In exploring her story, Rita realized she was becoming Consciously Competent— she was learning. It wasn't supposed to be easy or comfortable. Understanding this made it progressively easier for her to start opening up and implementing behavioral changes. She began to develop her own self-care plan. Shortly after, Rita came in looking particularly cheerful and confident. She told me, "After forty-three years of marriage, last night was the first time I ever said 'no' to my husband." She had come into the program being helpless and left an empowered woman.

CHAPTER 9

TROUBLESHOOTING: DIAGNOSING AND TREATING CHALLENGES

Diagnosing and treating challenges initially requires focus on the primary or internal level, which revolves around everything we've been discussing.

It took me years to understand this essential piece of the puzzle. I was consumed by solving one problem after another externally while ignoring what was happening internally. I was creating problems that didn't exist, except, of course, in my own mind.

"Problems" Often Vanish When We Start Looking Internally

We often delude ourselves into believing "If something external to me were different, I'd feel better." External factors certainly influence how we feel, but what happens when we become dependent on external conditions?

We are never truly satisfied. The relief we experience from improved (external) conditions does not last. We quickly want either **more** or something else to change, which leads to the next self-created problem that needs to be solved—an endless and frustrating process.

Understanding where we stand internally is essential. It enables us to access our intuitive nature (consciousness), which is our own personal "guru" that points us to the *correct action* at any given moment.

Regardless of the issue, the first step is *always* to go internally and find a sense of balance. Then, we can ask ourselves, "Is there any external action required at this moment?" (Tolle)

Remember, it is the intention behind our actions that determines the most important outcomes in life—how we feel about ourselves.

This is precisely why an inauthentic apology feels so empty. The same is true for any action taken from a place of fear, anxiety, or frustration. Even if we fix the problem, we experience the negative emotion generated by our actions.

Here's how I began to learn this valuable lesson.

Several years ago, I received an overpriced bill from my car insurance company. I immediately went into a reactive, downright nasty state and acted like a jerk to the customer service representative.

As it turned out, the company had made a mistake, and I was overcharged by several hundred dollars. Perhaps not so coincidentally, I had a call scheduled with my coach later that afternoon.

I'm embarrassed to admit that I was feeling somewhat satisfied (at least temporarily) with my ability to resolve the error. When I told Karin the story, she asked, "Do you really want to put that type of energy out into the world?"

The answer is obvious. I was not operating from my deepest intention at that moment, and my lack of internal focus was a catalyst for creating a great deal of negative energy. I could have resolved the billing error with no drama had I started internally first—recognizing my emotions and overreaction.

Instead, I projected the anger and frustration I was feeling onto the customer service representative who wasn't even at fault. I was more concerned about the result (getting my bill fixed now!) than remaining in a state of internal peace.

If I had been more aware at the time, my internal dialogue would have sounded like this: "This bill seems way too high, and I'm feeling angry that I have to deal with this now. Before I jump to any conclusions and assume they raised my rate, let me calm down and give them a call." I then would have proceeded to resolve the situation with a drama-free exchange.

I know this is so "duh" that it may seem superfluous to discuss, but the subtle ways we all fall into this sort of an emotionally triggered trap are not always so obvious.

It takes a great deal of courage and openness to discover our unique strategies for operating in this way, but it is well worth the effort.

That being said, challenges do arise in life that require attention and action on both the internal and external levels. Let's talk about the Troubleshooting Process that we can apply to these scenarios.

Troubleshooting in Action

Truthfully, I am not sure how to start this section, so let me use this very situation to demonstrate how I troubleshoot challenges.

"Problem": I don't know how to complete this section.

Internal Level Assessment: "I'm feeling anxiety because I believe I have to be perfect, and that I'm supposed to know how to do everything before I start. This is completely normal and something most authors experience. Judging myself for feeling this way isn't going to help.

What can I do to get calm and centered so I can express my ideas in the clearest and most concise way possible?"

<u>Internal Level Actions</u>: "I know breathing deeply, sensing the space in and around my body, and remembering my deepest intention help me remain calm and focused, so I'll do all of that for a few minutes before I continue." (This is *exactly* what I did before writing this "Troubleshooting in Action" section, which I didn't fully realize until I started writing.)

<u>External Level Assessment/Actions</u>: "Obviously this section isn't going to write itself, but I can start, now that I'm centered. What knowledge or experiences can I draw upon that might give me some direction? Eckhart Tolle recommends starting where you are in any given moment. So, rather than resisting this anxiety, I will allow it to be and see what happens." (This Troubleshooting Process is what came about after I took a little dose of my own medicine. Not bad, eh?)

<u>External Level Action (Involving Others)</u>: In this particular case, external action involving other people is not necessary. However, let's say that I was experiencing a serious writer's block and was really distressed. I may have proceeded in the following way: "Even though I know I have my own answers, I can't access them right now. I need to reach out for support to help me get some clarity. It may also be helpful to get some coaching about the writing process."

Troubleshooting the Top Seven Clinical Challenges

The process described above included scripts that may appear obvious on the surface, but it is only through deep personal exploration that this type of action becomes natural to implement.

One of my first clients said, "We all have our unique emotional hot spots," which is true. We have all experienced "troubleshooting" without giving it a second thought, but we also can feel completely lost when we are triggered emotionally. It is possible that the following examples may not specifically apply to you.

You may be saying, "Well, I already do this naturally, so it isn't something I need to learn or practice."

Yes, some people are more natural at this than others, but as my client pointed out, we each have our unique hot spots. So, even if these specific issues do not apply to you, I would recommend exploring areas in your life where you may be easily thrown off balance.

I am mentioning this because it is important that you create your own "process for the process." You must find a unique set of tools, thought patterns, and strategies that work for you. Trust your own wisdom. The examples I include can be a useful guide, but what is most important is to energetically align yourself with whatever words you choose.

By practicing what you are learning in this book, you will begin to express the most authentic version of yourself. It will not feel like a script; your words will flow from the core of your being, which will feel amazing.

Here are seven common opportunities ("problems") and ways these situations can be addressed using the process we have been discussing.

TOP SEVEN OPPORTUNITIES ("PROBLEMS")

1. "Problem": Performance anxiety and fear of failure.

    Internal Level Assessment: "I'm feeling really scared right

now, because I don't know what I'm doing. My clients are going to know that I'm clueless. I might even fail! I know I'll probably be fine, but it doesn't feel that way. I'm just not feeling very confident.

I have to remember, though, that these feelings are normal. Everyone experiences something like this. I must remember to allow these feelings to be—resisting them only makes them stronger. Besides, I'm not supposed to know everything. It's unreasonable to expect to be perfect from the start. What can I do right now to prepare myself to perform at my best?"

Internal Level Actions: "I know self-reflection like this makes me more relaxed and focused. Specifically, reviewing my deepest intentions also helps a great deal, so I am going to do that as much as possible. I also know that simply breathing properly keeps my body relaxed and out of a fight-or-flight mode."

External Level Assessment/Actions: "First, I'll keep my Deepest Intention list all over the place (phone, car, fridge, bathroom, etc.). I'll keep up my self-care practices (exercise, journaling, yoga, meditation, etc.) throughout my clinical; they will help keep me balanced. Reviewing my books and taking notes will also help me to be more prepared and feel more confident."

External Level Actions (Involving Others): "I will inform my supervisor of my preferred learning style and communicate openly and honestly from the start. It is important for me to let him or her know of any performance issues or concerns I may be having that require attention. If I don't let him or her know what is going on with me, I won't get the help I need, so it's up to me to communicate."

2. "Problem": I don't get along with my supervisor. *Side Note*: This problem often speaks to a larger issue. Ideally, all supervisors would be great role models, but sadly, this is not always the case. Some people in positions of authority (e.g., your supervisor) negatively impact the people they supervise by unconsciously identifying with their emotions. This puts the supervisee in an awkward position, especially when the supervisor's feelings are projected onto their student (i.e., "My student is so *frustrating!*"). Remember, this is *not* a personal or conscious process; they are *not* stopping and thinking about their actions. This situation, in fact, can also happen in reverse—where the student becomes the "projector."

Regardless of who is right and who is wrong, your job (as mine) is to **always** start by exploring your role in the conflict. Magical things can happen when we (either the supervisor or the student) focus on "being the change we want to see in the world" (Gandhi).

Internal Level Assessment: "I'm feeling really frustrated with my supervisor. We are clearly not on the same page. The way she communicates makes me feel really uncomfortable. I don't know how I'm going to get through this clinical, but I'd better start looking at what I can do differently. Blaming her for feeling this way, even if she is playing a bigger role, is only going to make things worse.

"I must allow myself to feel these feelings in order to give them a chance to pass. Then, instead of looking at the situation as a problem, I'm going use it as an opportunity to create a more solid personal boundary so that I will not be so easily influenced by her behavior. Besides, deep down I know she is not trying to be difficult. Compassion is a better option than judgment, both for her and me."

Internal Level Actions: "It is difficult to admit that the behaviors we judge in others are fragmented parts of our own personality that we have been denying. What is it about her that bothers me so much? I need to commit to looking internally at my reaction to something she says or does."

External Level Assessment/Actions: "The exercises that Dan recommended in Chapter 4 will help me tease out the qualities I have been denying. Exploring some of the resources, like *The Shadow Effect* and the TED Talk "The Power of Vulnerability," may also shed light on my role. As Dr. Joe teaches, the more we build a model and have a knowledge base that explains our behavior, the better we can use that information to create the best outcomes. I also need to keep track as I progress, so I will try the "Learning Journaling" exercise as well."

External Level Actions (Involving Others): "I must be able to effectively communicate with my supervisor to be successful, no matter how difficult he or she might be. So, I will do my best to be the bigger person and speak in a way that is authentic and assertive while at the same time respect his or her delicate sensibilities. I will focus on myself and say things like, 'Please let me know what I can do to be most successful.' I will also avoid using the word *you* to keep him or her from acting defensively. I know that focusing on my core will keep me really centered, and that in itself will point me to the right action in any given moment. I am confident that I can manage this situation on my own, but I know that I have the option to reach out for support (clinical coordinator, school director, personal therapist/coach, etc.) if necessary."

3. "Problem": I am having difficulty establishing rapport.

Internal Level Assessment: "I am feeling uncomfortable and having trouble connecting with my clients. I don't know how to relate to them. We have such different backgrounds, and many of them are facing challenges that seem insurmountable. I don't even know what I would do if I were in their shoes. I really want to help, but the more I try, the worse I do.

"I must start by acknowledging my feelings. This is a new experience, and I do not have to be perfect or be able to connect with everyone yet. I also *know* that I am not really trying when I am at my best, so I really need to practice getting out of my own way. I bet they are picking up the energy I project when I am too attached to the results and only want them to like me."

Internal Level Actions: "The self-reflection is helping me

see that I am clearly *not* operating from my deepest intention. My need to help and my wanting them to like me are causing me to restrain my authentic self. Finding a resource on the best way to establish rapport may give me some great ideas."

External Level Assessment/Actions: "Keeping my Deepest Intention list handy and practicing Segment Intention Setting (see page 90) before each session will make a big difference. I can also review my Three Most Important Things list and practice the Three Essentials for staying connected to my core. I bet that will go a long way toward establishing rapport as we gear up to connect on a deeper level."

External Level Actions (Involving Others): "I realize this problem is primarily internal, but asking my supervisor for specific feedback could make a big difference. The more I know what is working (or not), the more I can use this to my advantage. Asking my clients directly may also be a good idea. Questions like, 'What do you think went well today? What really worked for you? What could make it better next time?' would let them know that I care about their opinions, and I can use their feedback to improve the quality of my service."

4. "Problem": I do not like my placement.

Internal Level Assessment: "I am feeling really frustrated about my placement. I have *no* interest in working with this population, and I made that very clear to my school. Now, I have to be here for 12 weeks, and I am *not* happy.

"I must start by acknowledging my feelings. This is not about being happy all the time. It is about accepting "what is" and doing the best I can. Fighting the fact that I am here is only going to make things more difficult."

Internal Level Actions: "I am going to have to keep my inner dog on a short leash—meaning I will really have to pay attention. Even though this is not my ideal placement, I realize that being present is the only thing that offers long-term satisfaction. I will review my deepest intentions and pay attention to my senses, which will help me stay clear and focused. I want to perform my best, even though I would rather be somewhere else."

External Level Assessment/Actions: "The more I can focus on doing the best job I can, the better I will feel. Instead of complaining to myself about being here, I will see what I can learn about this population. I will check out some resources and make sure to give everyone my fullest attention. Who knows, maybe I will be surprised and end up liking it here."

External Level Actions (Involving Others): "I realize this problem is primarily internal, so I don't think I need to involve my supervisor. Even though this placement is not my choice, I must do my very best. I am going to get out of my comfort zone and really get to know my colleagues and clients. Many of them are passionate about being here, and I bet I can learn a lot from them. I am going to take my focus off of me and do the best job I can."

5. "Problem": I just want to graduate.

    Internal Level Assessment: "I am so *done* with school and I don't want to be here. I already have my job lined up, and now I have to spend a lot of time working for free.

    "I better fully accept that I am here or I could really get myself into trouble."

    *****I have witnessed one capable student failing for this reason.*****

    Internal Level Actions: "I must accept 'what is' on a global (length of placement) and moment-by-moment basis. I could really screw things up if I let my inner dog race to the finish line."

    External Level Assessment/Actions: "It may be helpful to review the chapter on acceptance and to complete some of the exercises. Feeling excited about graduation is completely normal, so I do need to be compassionate with myself. But I also need to remember that the clients and colleagues that I am working with deserve my full attention. If I don't fully accept that I am going to be here for a while, they will *know* it, and it will impact my performance. I don't want to make that mistake."

    External Level Actions (Involving Others): "My ego is telling me my life is going to be *so* much better after I graduate. I know it will feel great, but that feeling won't last very long. Paying attention to the present moment is the only thing that offers long-term satisfaction. So, I am going to keep my 'senior-itis' in check and give everyone my full attention. I will feel better for it and will perform at my best."

6. "Problem:" I am not comfortable with this type of client.

Internal Level Assessment: "I wish I didn't feel this way, but I am not comfortable with this person. I don't understand his lifestyle, and we have nothing in common. I know I am being judgmental, but it is part of human nature to feel this way—it does not make me a bad person.

"I must allow myself to feel these feelings. Then, I can rise above them and do the best job I can. Focusing on what I can learn about myself will make me feel better and might even result in discovering that we have some things in common."

Internal Level Actions: "I remember learning that 'the world is our mirror,' so what is it about this person that rubs me the wrong way? I don't like the client's lifestyle choices (e.g., substance abuse, poor diet, etc.). Even though I am not a substance abuser, I am definitely guilty of having inadequate self-control and have addictive issues like overeating and checking my phone too often. The client is also kind of 'blah' and I know how that feels. I am really going to start paying attention when I am feeling triggered, and ask the question, 'What is it about **me** that is making me feel this way?' "

External Level Assessment/Actions: "I am going to 'scan for viruses' and do some of the upgrading software exercises to program myself to be successful with him. I will learn something about myself instead of feeling stressed about having to work with this person."

External Level Actions (Involving Others): "Now that I am focusing on myself, I am in a better position to get creative when working with him. Focusing on getting the client to participate in the treatment has not been working, so what else can I do? I can ask my supervisor for some suggestions. Maybe I can find out what this client is passionate about and connect on that level. Perhaps I can learn about this person's musical interests and incorporate that into our sessions. I could also just be really honest (i.e., "The Power of Vulnerability") and remind the client that I am new to all this and still learning, and that it would be helpful if he could let me know how I could best be of service (making sure to maintain friendly professional boundaries, of course). I am not certain if any of these strategies will work but I will feel better doing my best to create a healthy therapeutic relationship."

7. "Problem": I am not comfortable taking a leadership/ authoritative role.

Internal Level Assessment: "I am uncomfortable being an authority figure to my clients. I am so much younger, and I don't want to be disrespectful. It feels like they are sensing my weakness and that I am not guiding them properly. Truthfully, I am more concerned about them liking me than I am about providing the best care. I don't think I trust myself (who am I to be doing this?), and I'm trying to deny this feeling.

"I must start by accepting 'what is' ("I am not being professional enough") and developing the skill of being an authority figure but in a balanced way. I am not doing my clients any favor by being like this, so it is time for me to change this pattern."

Internal Level Actions: "Paying attention to my breathing will help me stay calmer and accept my emotions as they arise. This is about me; it is not what the client is doing that is making me uncomfortable. This person is just bringing out the insecurity that is already within me. This is a great opportunity for me to grow beyond this limitation. My deepest intention is to be a role model. The more I remind myself of this truth, the better I will be able to connect and serve."

External Level Assessment/Actions: "Like an athlete warming up, I am going to have to mentally and physically prepare myself before work. It does not have to take long— just a minute or two can make a big difference. First, I will center myself by 'feeling I,' and then I will review my deepest intentions right before the session. Emotions may come up throughout the day, but this will go a long way to helping me be prepared."

External Level Actions (Involving Others): "I have enabled my client to run the session by not being an assertive professional. It is time for me to set better boundaries. I already feel more empowered after processing everything in this way, but it may also be helpful to have a conversation with the client in order to set a better tone for our therapeutic relationship. I will have to stay present to know what to say, but I can imagine it will sound something like this:

"'I appreciate your willingness to work with me, but it is important that we understand our roles as we move forward. You are the client, and your opinions matter very much to me, but I have gone to great lengths to educate myself on how to treat a person with your condition. So it is important for you to respect my area of expertise. I am confident that we can find a common ground and work more effectively if we both respect each other's roles.'"

Guiding Questions

You may find the following questions helpful in working your way through the process.

Internal Level Assessment: What am I feeling? What feelings might I be resisting? What is my intention in this moment? What is my deepest intention?

Internal Level Actions: What helps me get centered? What have I learned that might be helpful in this situation?

External Level Assessment/Actions: Is there any exercise or technique I can use? What might help this situation?

External Level Actions (Involving Others): Am I doing everything I can on my end? What may happen if I don't bring this up with the other person? Is this the right action, even if they do not respond as I would like them to?

Summary

Each of the examples included in this chapter follow the same formula and draw from specific areas of knowledge covered in this book. Ironically, when we are truly present we don't need this type of guide—the process happens naturally.

Staying present and looking internally is what gives us access to our greatest intelligence, empowering us to effortlessly troubleshoot the challenges we face in life. But until we have all become Zen masters, little road maps like these can be very helpful.

I wish you the best of luck with your clinical rotations. Please join our growing community at www.daneisnerconsulting.com for ongoing support as you embark on your career in healthcare.

Troubleshooting Leads to Success

Years ago, we had a student who didn't like her placement. She looked downright miserable, and if her performance did not improve, she was at risk of failing. It had nothing to do with her intelligence or clinical reasoning. It had EVERYTHING to do with her attitude.

About halfway through her clinical, she attended my in-service that summarizes the importance of *presence* and teaches how to apply oneself therapeutically.

When I asked her what she had learned, she replied, "I'm never present, not even with my (one-year-old) daughter." This took a great deal of honesty and courage. I believe it was the catalyst that dramatically improved her performance. As you may recall, acceptance (i.e., "Yes, I am never present.") is a precursor to change.

A few days later, two of my colleagues told me, "Oh my God, Dan, you should have seen her. She was so in the zone running her group today!" The interesting thing was that the student didn't think the group went very well.

Why?

It did not go as she expected. She had planned out the treatment but for a variety of reasons (not necessarily her fault) it just wasn't working. However, instead of going into panic mode and trying harder, she remained focused and present. This gave her access to her greater intuitive intelligence, which enabled her to effortlessly adapt (in the moment) to best meet the needs of her clients.

That day, she provided treatment like a seasoned professional. However, it wasn't until we processed (examined after the session) that she understood what she did to optimize her performance.

Her supervisor later told me how her performance consistently improved following that experience. Understanding how to troubleshoot issues like "I don't want to be here" is both personally and professionally empowering.

ACKNOWLEDGEMENTS

Honestly, there isn't enough room in this entire book to acknowledge all of those who have influenced me.

If you don't hear yourself personally mentioned, please know that it is in no way an indication of the significance of your impact. You all have touched my heart in some unique way.

First, I'd like to thank my mom and dad for their unconditional love and support. This book would not have been possible without the positive influence you've both had on my life. I'd also like to thank Dad for being my unofficial editor. You really helped my writing to become more clear and concise.

I'd like to express my gratitude to my boss Lila. You have allowed me the freedom to "research" and test out the ideas in this book over the last nine years. The simple but powerful formula I have created would not have been possible had you not gone out of your way to provide me with opportunities to expand professionally.

Thank you to so many of my colleagues (some of whom you have met here) who have had the willingness to embrace the wisdom discussed in this book. Your stories have inspired me to get my message out to the world.

I'd also like to thank my coach Karin, and my friend and mentor Karl for being wonderful role models. You have both inspired me in ways that cannot be expressed with words. The same is true for my "Spiritual Partners" Jen and Laura, not to mention all my friends in the Dr. Joe community.

I'd like to acknowledge my editors, Pam and Sally, and my graphic designer, Jason. Pam, thank you for allowing me the freedom to find my own voice. Sally, thank you for your meticulous fine-tuning and polishing. Jason, the images you created simplify the teaching beautifully.

And I would like to personally thank a few of the many authors and teachers who have heavily impacted the creation of this formula. Dr. Joe Dispenza, Dr. Les Fehmi, Eckhart Tolle, Tara Brach, Brené Brown, and the late Debbie Ford—thank you for the work that you do.

Finally, I'd like to thank you for your willingness to explore the ideas discussed in this book. You inspire me to continue to express my passion and to provide the highest quality of care.

BIBLIOGRAPHY & RECOMMENDED RESOURCES

Books

Brach, Tara. *Radical Acceptance: Embracing Your Life With the Heart of a Buddha*. New York: Bantam, 2003.

Brown, Brené. *Daring Greatly: How the Courage to Be Vulnerable Transforms the Way We Live, Love, Parent, and Lead*. New York: Portfolio Penguin, 2013.

Chopra, Deepak. *The Seven Spiritual Laws of Success: A Practical Guide to the Fulfillment of Your Dreams*. Novato, CA: New World Library/ Amber-Allen, 1994.

Covey, Stephen R. *The 7 Habits of Highly Effective People*. New York: Simon & Schuster, 2013.

Dispenza, Joe. *Breaking the Habit of Being Yourself: How to Lose Your Mind and Create a New One*. Carlsbad: Hay House, 2012.

———. *Evolve Your Brain: The Science of Changing Your Mind*. Deerfield Beach, FL: HCI, 2008.

———. *You Are the Placebo: Making Your Mind Matter*. Carlsbad: Hay House, 2014

Fehmi, Les, and Jim Robbins. *The Open-Focus Brain: Harnessing the Power of Attention to Heal Mind and Body*. Boulder: Trumpeter Books, 2008.

Ford, Deborah. *The Dark Side of Light Chasers*. New York: Riverhead Trade, 1998.

Hicks, Esther, and Jerry Hicks. *The Law of Attraction: The Basics of the Teachings of Abraham*. Carlsbad: Hay House, 2006.

Lesser, Elizabeth. *Broken Open: How Difficult Times Can Help Us Grow.* New York: Villard, 2003.

Lipton, Bruce H. *The Biology of Belief: Unleashing the Power of Consciousness, Matter, & Miracles.* Carlsbad: Hay House, 2007.

Pert, Candace B. *Molecules of Emotion: The Science Behind Mind-Body Medicine.* New York: Simon & Schuster, 1999.

Ramtha. *Ramtha: The White Book.* Yelm, WA: JZK Publishing, 2005.

Schucman, Helen. *A Course In Miracles, Combined Volume, 3rd Ed.* Mill Valley: Foundation for Inner Peace, 2008.

Tolle, Eckhart. *A New Earth: Awakening to Your Life's Purpose.* New York: Penguin, 2007.

———. *The Power of Now: A Guide to Spiritual Enlightenment.* Novato, CA: New World Library, 1999.

Film/Video

Musical Prescriptions for Health, DVD. Directed by Barry Goldstein. Yelm, WA: Encephalon, 2014

The Shadow Effect: Illuminating the Hidden Power of Your True Self, DVD. Directed by Scott Cervine. Carlsbad, CA: Debbie Ford Films and Hay House, Inc., 2009

What the Bleep Do We Know!?, DVD. Directed by Betsy Chasse, Mark Vicente, and William Arntz. Los Angeles, CA: 20th Century Fox, 2005

Brown, Brené. "Listening to Shame." Filmed March 2012. TED video, 20:38. Posted March 2012. https://www.ted.com/talks/brene_brown_listening_to_shame?language=en

———. "The Power of Vulnerability." Filmed June 2010. TED video, 20:19. Posted December 2010. https://www.ted.com/talks/brene_brown_on_vulnerability?language=en

ABOUT THE AUTHOR

Dan Eisner is a Psychiatric Occupational Therapist and Certified Life Coach with over 18 years experience. He specializes in the development of Mindfulness & Emotional Intelligence, using principles based on the latest advances in neuroscience. While Dan is passionate about many things, what he loves the most is inspiring others to trust their intuition and to stay on their own path. He works wisely to be the best role model of what he teaches, with the intention of helping himself and others discover more peace and joy in life.

Dan lives and works in Baltimore, Maryland. He loves all animals and considers his two dog-like cats, Freddie and Muka, to be his furry children. Dan's an avid golfer and poker player, and also enjoys more adventurous activities like skiing and SCUBA diving.

Visit his website:

www.DanEisnerConsulting.com

CPSIA information can be obtained
at www.ICGtesting.com
Printed in the USA
LVHW080352300519
619544LV00006B/7/P